FREEING
THE
UNLOVED
GIRL

A WOMAN'S GUIDE TO HEALING FROM
CHILDHOOD ABUSE AND
CONDITIONING

MARISA RUSSO

First Print Edition: Nov, 2015   First eBook Edition: Nov, 2015
ISBN: 978-0-9875172-8-9   ISBN: 978-0-9944798-0-8

While the author has made every effort to provide accurate internet addresses and other contact information at the time of publication, the author does not assume any responsibility for errors, or for changes that occur after publication. Further, the author does not assume any responsibility for any related or third-party web sites or their content.

Disclaimer:
The author of this book does not dispense medical advice nor prescribe the use of any technique as a form of treatment for physical or medical problems without the advice of a physician, either directly or indirectly. The intent of the author is only to offer information of a general nature to help you in your quest for physical fitness and good health. In the event you use any of the information in this book for yourself, which is your constitutional right, the author and the publisher assume no responsibility for your actions.

EDITORS
Bryony Sutherland
Conna Craig
Cindy Dockendorff
Belinda McShane
Forensic Healing team

COVER DESIGNER
Andreea Vraciu

BOOK DESIGNER
iPublicidades

DEDICATION

My Forensic Healing sisters who continue to change lives
in every corner of our ever-changing world.

I was born innocent, pure, and free
And then my father took that away from me
As he inflicted abuse with anger and hate
He grabbed the belt; it was my fate
I was in a battlefield, I was in a war
He beat me
He molested me
He was the law
Every day I pleaded to God to take away the pain
But he never did, it was always the same

After one day of horror I shut myself down
I put on a happy face and became a clown
I said, "This is not happening." I pretended it was fine
I was frozen in pain; I was frozen in time
Life had no meaning; it was wasting away
I was living in fear and living in vain

As I peeled off the layers, I remembered the pain
I dropped to my knees, begging God to end it again
It was in those darkest moments that I connected to source
I found my gift, I found my force

Now I am whole I can help others heal
I finally know what it means to be real

Marisa Russo

ABOUT THE BOOK

Freeing the Unloved Girl is a woman's guide to healing from childhood abuse and conditioning.

"As parts of my childhood memories returned, I tried to make sense of it all. There were many pieces of the puzzle that started to come together as I retraced my steps. It started to make sense why I experienced high levels of anxiety, panic attacks, felt unsafe, and wanted to lock my bedroom door at night."

Abused as a child, Marisa Russo feared commitment and fell into a lifestyle of poor choices and negativity. Finally able to reclaim her true identity in her forties, she made it her life's work to help others in the same predicament. Having founded Forensic Healing, Marisa's investigative style of therapy first attracted praise in her book, **Women Breaking Free.** In this new offering, **Freeing the Unloved Girl,** Marisa helps readers discover and heal past hurts using a combination of examples and exercises, alongside words of encouragement and validation.

WHAT YOU WILL LEARN

A step-by-step liberating process of self-discovery and empowerment to;

- Remove the effects of emotional and physical abuse along with subtle and obvious conditioning from the stereotypes of being a woman.

- Reconnect to your ability as a woman to feel and know answers, solutions, and guidance that direct you to safety, truth and empowerment.

- Release guilt, negative associations and crippling preconceptions.

- Express yourself fully and feel free to be you, using conversation and expression analysis.

- Rate your relationships using the Positive Energy Index to enhance your personal power network.

- Live a proven, daily system to create a richer, more rewarding, and happier life.

ABOUT THE AUTHOR

An international award-winning teacher, author, speaker and healer, for twenty-five years Marisa Russo has been changing lives. With her Forensic Healing approach to therapy, the media refer to Marisa as the 'Sherlock Holmes of Healing'.

Marisa has a mind that never stops questioning, digging for answers and solutions. She thrives on solving the most challenging health conditions and life circumstances. After working with thousands of clients over the last two and a half decades, Marisa knows the mindset, the healing processes and techniques that really work to help people heal.

But it wasn't always this way for Marisa…

"I didn't always want to be an alternative therapist. In fact, I wasn't sure I'd amount to anything. I was 40 before I had the first, genuine liberating thought that I might actually have something to contribute to the world!

I was emotionally, physically and sexually abused as a child. I grew up feeling worthless and alone. A raft of addictions masked my pain. I was totally dysfunctional. My body and emotions were riddled with so much suffering that life seemed futile and death a welcome option.

For many years I travelled the globe, desperate to overcome and escape the chronic pain, fatigue, addictions and illnesses that resulted from years of abuse. The unrelenting pain led me to seek alternative therapy only because traditional doctors said I would have to live with the pain for the rest of my life – a prophecy that I wasn't about to accept!"

Marisa tried many different therapies and studied more than 60 courses. $310,000 later she discovered her healing gift. Through clearing her own condition, her energetic connection had grown so strong that she could read a person's body to accurately determine the cause of their condition and know how to bring relief.

In 2011, after many requests from clients to learn her methods, Marisa combined all of the alternative healing techniques she discovered into the Forensic Healing home-based and live training courses.

FREE COMPANION RESOURCE

Freeing Women Activation
The healing activation reverses the control and programmed
manipulations placed on women.

Use this link below to get free access:
http://marisarusso.com/fug-reader/

CONTENTS

CHAPTER 1
BREAKING POINT

"Is it just me or does everyone reach a breaking point in their life?

I couldn't understand why I suddenly burst into tears as I began my 8.00 a.m. shift at work. I enjoyed my job, my colleagues were nice, and everything had been fine the day before. I wasn't crying over a breakup, I didn't have a boyfriend at the time and even if that had been the case, I would've been cursing and wishing I'd never met him. But here I was, hiding behind my hands, unable to find a single reason for the uncontrollable tears that were making my body shake. I later realised it was the long overdue opening of Pandora's Box which, although I resisted with all my might, would never be closed again.

Only hours before, I had routinely gotten out of bed, eaten breakfast, and driven to work. Now, I couldn't even talk as the emotions poured out of me. My mind flashed back to my thirtieth birthday party two weeks earlier, when I had indulged myself and thrown a traditional ball with a Cinderella theme. I rented an outrageously elaborate pink ball gown, got some friends to dress up as footmen, and danced the night away. Hang the expenses — I wanted a fairy-tale evening of wishful thinking. I'd decided on Cinderella, as she had a happy ending to a miserable life. Now that's a clue right there! Having begun my thirtieth year with the promise of a great decade ahead, I thought I was happy — or at least, there was nothing discernibly making me unhappy.

Thank God there was no one in the reception room when I broke down. My job was answering incoming calls at the British Petroleum head office. The next co-worker would arrive at 9.00 a.m., so I had one hour to pull myself together before anyone witnessed what a basket case I had become. I felt like an overstuffed suitcase on its way home from an overindulgent shopping holiday: everything spills out as you push and squeeze the contents tightly into the case, trying to close the zipper without breaking it. It was obvious: my zipper was busted and could no longer hold the contents.

Despite the spillage, my mindset wasn't to take the day off and go home. I was a hard worker who always arrived early and stayed late. Time off had never been an option for me. My only choice was to soldier on and get the job done, just as I'd been doing my whole life. My emotions were pushed down and buried — not honoured, explored, or considered.

I couldn't leave my desk to go to the ladies' room, so I dug into my handbag for tissues and a compact mirror. As I looked into it, the reflection looking back could have easily been mistaken for someone the morning after a heavy night on the town. I closed the compact to avoid looking into my own eyes. I just hoped all the redness and swelling would be gone before anyone walked through the door.

Little did I know this was the beginning of an awakening process that would completely release me from my secret life of unspoken misery. Like the overstuffed suitcase, I was too full to notice what was inside and I purposely avoided looking within by creating days full of people to see and things to do. I was constantly rushing from one event to the next. I signed up for every available committee that would have me. I was dedicated to creating a life of constant distractions, so that I never had the time to be still and take a good look at myself.

A few years prior to this unravelling, I had travelled the world, searching for something that I felt was missing in my life. I had left my home in Australia and moved to Italy in my early twenties, where I almost married a handsome Florentine doctor named Marco, just after I joined the Mormon Church. After deciding not to marry him (more about my lunatic behaviour later), I returned to Melbourne and began working for British Petroleum. This is where the repressed contents of my past began spilling out. Nothing I tried could close the zipper on that bulging suitcase of emotions.

I had lived my life as a good citizen. While studying part-time for a health science degree, I was heavily involved in serving others through church callings. I worked hard to give myself a sense of being useful in the world. Yet all my life, my father's words continued to haunt me: "You're stupid. You're an idiot and you will never amount to anything." I was determined to prove him wrong and banish the damning judgement that echoed in my head.

By the time my thirties rolled around, I was struggling with chronic neck pain after a series of whiplash injuries. I spent a small fortune on traditional therapies that offered only temporary relief. Life continued on autopilot. I was like the robot on the TV series *Lost in Space*, repeating, "Danger, Will Robinson!" and ensuring that everyone else was taken care of, without ever considering myself. My automated response to addressing my own needs was: "That does not compute."

Putting other people's needs before my own seemed like the right thing to do. It was my way of being selfless and, therefore, worthy. I lived my life as most women do, believing my *self-worth* was associated with how *selfless* and giving I was to others.

My unexpected crying episode forced me to stop and reflect on my life. I began to realise that I had never felt fulfilled or good enough. Because of that, I attracted people who manipulated and took advantage of me. They reinforced the unworthiness I'd felt since my childhood. I had to finally acknowledge the physical, emotional, and sexual abuse my father had inflicted on me, instilling so much self-hatred that my body was reacting. At last, I was required to change, as the pain was too great to bear. Although I couldn't imagine it at the time, the long process of healing and changing eventually became a precious gift I could share with other women.

Since then, I have earned my black belt in self-respect. I have opened up to an ability to intuit others' agendas and intentions. I can feel and read people's energy fields allowing me to assist in clearing the energy blockages that are preventing them obtaining the same freedom and happiness I have finally gained in my own life.

TIME TO GET REAL

As you read this book, you might not yet know what's stopping your success or happiness. You might not be as deep in denial as I was! Maybe, for you, there's just a vague feeling that something isn't right, and you want to change. That's great, because even though it's a cliché, the first step to healing is admitting there's a problem.

This book will help you identify and work through emotional blocks of all kinds. After two decades of working with thousands of women from all over the world, it seems that in almost every case, women tend to relive relationship dynamics from their past — usually from childhood. The cycle of living and reliving the same pattern prevents them from moving forward. For some there's a specific traumatic event that has been suppressed or erased from their memory as a way to cope with the pain.

That is what happened to me. For others, it's subtler, less obvious, yet can be just as damaging with their experiences continually conditioning them, reinforcing feelings of guilt, shame, and low self-worth. This makes it a lot harder to see the dysfunction, as it's not so easy to pinpoint one specific event as the cause. It becomes a normal way of life, unless or until someone like me explains how a person's childhood needs were unmet.

No one ever knew what happened to me when I was a child. Even I was in denial about the abuse until my thirties. I had completely blocked out sections of my childhood so I could survive what felt like a living hell. As an adult, I became so adept at hiding my emotions that my body began to create inescapable physical pain. It was a desperate cry for help.

I eventually learned that my survival technique of shutting down my feelings was a very common reaction to trauma. If you experience sexual, emotional, or physical abuse, you learn to block your feelings in order to survive. It's not something that happens only with abuse. If you experience violence, war, life-changing accidents, sickness, ongoing stress, emotional neglect, homelessness, or severe economic distress, you learn to toughen up and switch off your emotions in order to cope. This can literally save your life at the time, but if the emotions aren't released, they will eventually cause emotional and physical dysfunction in your life.

SHORT-TERM GAIN, LONG-TERM LOSS

Women raised in a dysfunctional environment become accustomed to disassociating from their feelings and blocking out their past. Carried into adulthood, this survival technique can manifest as anxiety, depression, and fear. Most of the time, the cause isn't obvious. Even women who haven't experienced overt abuse are often faced with neglect from their parents, perhaps because male siblings were favoured, or their parents divorced or became otherwise unavailable, or for other reasons that may even have seemed insignificant at the time. There is a culture that expects women to care for everyone around them without acknowledging their own needs. This makes it difficult to identify the reasons they don't experience fulfilling relationships and career success later in life.

Over years of working with women, I began to see consistent patterns. If you're reading this, and relate to the difficulty of living as your true self, rest assured — you're in good company. The struggle to be acknowledged, valued, and respected for living as your true self and following your heart is something many women must overcome. You get through it by reclaiming your power, and giving yourself the freedom to follow your own inner guidance, or what I refer to as your personal GPS.

Like so many women, by the time I reached my thirties, the stress of living a disconnected life finally caught up with me. I couldn't spend one moment longer pretending everything was okay. Something in me had to change.

Even though I had travelled the world and lived in some amazing countries, I was unhappy. I pretended to lead a normal life, but underneath, I knew something wasn't right. I had a secret wish whenever I came to a red *EXIT* sign in a public building. I'd pray the door would be the exit from my suffering. Whenever I walked through, I looked up at the God I had always known, the one I believed held all the power, and I felt great dismay that I found myself still living in pain on the other side of the *EXIT* sign.

Realising I needed to change was the first step toward healing in my life. It took time to peel off the layers, but eventually I regained enough strength to face the pain of the abuse. True healing occurred when my body and mind were strong enough to deal with my past. I worked for years with many therapists and healers and attended numerous courses to heal myself and develop my own intuitive and healing abilities. Gradually, I was able to unlock my gift and heal myself. This experience taught me how to connect and heal women with similar issues. My mission is to enable all women to experience freedom, empowerment, and equality and find their worth through healing from abuse, trauma, judgment, and conditioning.

The most important aspect of healing is the process of reconnecting with yourself. To begin, you must rediscover your trust in the universe, and then surrender, and let go. The prospect of losing control may resurrect fear, anxiety, or other emotions from your childhood. Trust in the process of receiving healing. Use the knowledge I have gained, and apply the methods throughout these chapters, by completing the

25 steps that have been extracted from the Freeing Women's workshop I conduct. You will be gently led to where you need to be. Surrender and allow yourself to be guided; everything will work out. The universe will orchestrate a journey for you to heal.

SOURCING THE POWER TO HEAL

In an attempt to heal or find yourself, have you searched for answers in books, workshops, or meditation retreats yet still felt something was missing? This is why I developed the Forensic Healing System (http://forensichealing.com). It is an alternative therapy healing system that finds the cause of the negative condition and releases it. By breaking down the walls and façades you've built up over the years, it reveals and frees your true self in a way that can't be found elsewhere.

So, what exactly is your true or authentic self? It's who you'd be if you didn't spend your time trying to be what others want you to be, trying to be who you think you should be, who you must, or ought to be. It's who you'd be if you knew that it's okay to discover what you want in life and go after it. In fact, it's more than okay: it's your birthright!

Women have been told countless times and in countless ways that it's selfish to be who they really are, to take care of themselves, and go after what they desire. The truth is that the world needs strong, powerful, vibrant women who are living passionately.

Think about it: who is most likely to bring about positive change in the world: a shy, timid, scared woman, or a strong, powerful, passionate woman? Think of the women you admire the most. Would you like to be more like them? Read on!

I imagine that reading this book isn't your first attempt at change? Many times over the years I've heard women say, "I thought I was over this. I thought I'd already dealt with this, so why does it keep coming up?" I wrote this book to honour your persistence and let you know there is a way out of the darkness.

To thrive in spite of a painful past, you need to access your inner power and strength you probably don't know you possess. This exists inside you, right now. It's the power and strength that comes from survival. It's true what they say: what doesn't kill you makes you stronger. Your past has stretched and moulded you. This book will take you on a journey to transform those painful experiences into freedom and power. These attributes will then become a source of strength that can be used to help achieve whatever you desire.

BARE YOUR SCARS

Your past no longer provides an excuse to be a victim. It's not going to stop you from reaching your greatness. Similar to a physical scar, your past is part of you. Instead of hiding it away and feeling ashamed, you can reveal its truth. Allow your scars to be seen. No more secrets or hiding your pain and feelings. You will be proud of your scars!

Feel strengthened and empowered because you survived. You are stronger than you realise, and your story is one of triumph and freedom. You are finally going to *transform your pain into your power*. You will begin to understand how truly resilient you are. I've learned over years of working with therapists and listening to my own intuition that true healing and transformation only occur when you've completely freed yourself from past conditioning and the experiences that led you to live only half a life.

As you read on, you'll begin to understand how deeply my own history of abuse was buried. You'll understand why it took me so many years to get to the root of the issue and then, finally, regain my power. You'll also understand why I've dedicated my life to helping other women become free from crippling, chronic pain and unhappiness. In my story, you may see parts of yourself. It is my hope that you'll feel inspired by how my life changed once I gained self-worth and became empowered.

It's your birthright to live your best, most authentic life! You can achieve the freedom and happiness that comes from living in integrity, from living passionately and following your own path. From never again allowing yourself to be controlled by others or by what has been done to you.

Before we get started, I acknowledge the amount of strength, determination, and honesty it takes to heal. I admire your courage for choosing this path. What I bring to the table is the ability to connect with your energy field, in order to help you reconnect with the essence of who you are. You might call this your spiritual force, your authentic self, or your soul. My journey has allowed me to feel energy from others, and connect to their feelings. This ability has given me deep insights on how to identify the individual needs for each woman to heal.

THE MAGIC OF BEING CONNECTED

Two of the most remarkable outcomes as you embark on this journey are that the magic returns and doors begin to open to great opportunities. When you connect to the inner power that's available to you, you'll become unstoppable. Once you get a taste of this freedom and empowerment, you'll never go back. Your eyes will reclaim their original sparkle as they express the joy that radiates from a soaring soul.

A while ago, I was surprised by such a transformation and it still touches my heart to this day. It was relatively early in my healing career that I was invited to speak at various locations in the United States. It was my first American healing tour and I was still unsure of my gift and myself. I saw myself as an Australian jumping out of my little fish bowl and diving into the big, wide ocean of the USA! I wasn't even sure anyone would turn up to see me demonstrate my healing abilities.

Americans had never met me, so I struggled to see how the tour would be successful. By that time I was married to my then-husband, John, a man who trusted in my gift enough to invest his precious time and our entire life savings to help me reach a wider audience.

John had a sharp business sense and shared my ability to read people and situations. From the moment we met, ours was a natural partnership. His business acumen complemented my healing goals, and we formed a team to expand my workshop capacity and produce online programs for women around the world. I went along with his plans for a US tour despite my initial reluctance.

Even though I trusted this was the next logical step, when the tour finally began, I remained sceptical. I spent the first week touring Los Angeles, and was pleasantly surprised by the encouraging number of people who attended the demonstrations. Slowly, my confidence grew as I received positive feedback. The event organisers and audiences were all very kind and open to my message. Still, I wasn't quite sure whether I was making an impact.

Sunday was my first free day, so John and I decided to attend one of Reverend Michael Bernard Beckwith's presentations at his Agape International Spiritual Center in Los Angeles. There, he delivers his message of hope and empowerment. Over the years, his following has grown to millions worldwide. I had seen his interview segments in the film *The Secret* many times and his message resonated deeply with me. In the film, he says that when we understand and apply the timeless laws of the universe, we can create anything we desire. If we believe in something, visualise it, and move towards it with confidence, it cannot help but show up.

That day, Michael conducted three sessions to over six thousand people. The audience members patiently lined up outside the centre before each session, anticipating Michael's message of reclaiming power and hope. When our group was ushered in, we could feel the energy buzzing with good vibes. We arrived early, so we found seats close to the stage. When I looked at the row in front of me, I noticed the famous singer Chaka Khan.

What are the odds? I thought. This must be a good omen!

As the event began, Michael's wife Rickie Byars-Beckwith sang and I immediately felt a deep, warm love embrace me. I watched the close-up of her angelic face on the big screen above the stage, her smile lighting up the entire auditorium. Rickie sang from her heart and my body relaxed as the emotions I was feeling moved me to tears.

It is a feeling similar to when you hold a newborn baby and sense that innocent connection of love. You are drawn in and know that you are in the presence of something sacred. The baby is your only focus, as your spirit reminds you how pure love can feel. Time stands still in such precious moments and I truly felt filled with gratitude for the musical experience I would never forget.

I don't know if I was the only one with tears rolling down my cheeks, but I completely forgot where I was for the entire time she sang. When Rickie finished, Michael appeared on stage. I was excited to see him in the flesh and experience the magnetic presence that so many had talked about; indeed, I sensed his connection to something greater.

Michael looked out across the audience and began acknowledging and introducing the many famous people in his congregation. I felt a crazy impulse to connect with him.

In my mind, I found myself shouting, *Pick me, pick me, Michael!*

As soon as the thought appeared, Michael pointed directly at me.

"Weren't you at the Bodhi Tree yesterday?" My heart nearly stopped! He smiled at me and continued, "I saw the light above your head and I heard about your amazing healings; I knew it was you."

For a moment, I thought I had literally yelled out "Pick me!" and Michael was humouring me. *How embarrassing*, I muttered to myself as I lowered my head. Then I realised this couldn't be the reason he'd identified me as John would have given me a hard jab if I did call out. I surmised that one of Michael's staff members must have attended the healing demonstration I gave at the Bodhi Tree Bookstore in LA and told him. He then used some other intuitive ability to identify me.

It was such a surreal moment. It was as if he read my mind, and politely responded to my crazy plea. But the connection was not to end there, for Michael then motioned me to join him on the stage! In seconds, a kind gentleman came to my side, took me by the arm, and guided me to the steps. My tour publicist, Dawna Shuman, quickly grabbed my itinerary from her bag and handed it to Michael.

As he looked over it, Michael read off my tour dates to the audience, and handed the stage to me so I could say a few words. I was speechless. Nobody had prepared me for that moment. Never in my wildest imagination did I believe I would share a stage with Reverend Michael Beckwith. My mind went blank.

What do I say? I stumbled through a few remarks, being mindful that he had given some of his precious audience time to me, then looked over to him to indicate that I had finished. To this day, when I review the video footage, it still surprises me that I got anything out at all. Next time you hear the adage, "Ask and ye shall receive," remember to be prepared to receive!

Since then, I have become more comfortable with who I am and my abilities as a healer and speaker. I have completed many more tours, workshops, and TV interviews. If I were called on stage again today, I'm sure I would feel less like a deer in headlights. My confidence has grown, as the conviction of my mission has been etched into every cell in my body.

ARE YOU READY TO FACE WHAT LIES WITHIN?

The moral of this story goes beyond just getting what you ask for. It's about understanding that life is an ongoing journey for you to reach your greatness. You may feel you've already attended every workshop and read every book; you may feel you're still not there. Remember you are growing and learning with each new experience. It's all part of your process. You have the ability to reach a confident, empowered place in your life, and to achieve everything you've ever wanted. What you are currently experiencing in your life is a gauge of your level of emotional and spiritual balance.

When you get called to your stage — or whatever that may be for you — know that you deserve to be there. The key to getting there lies in undoing the past by examining the experiences that created the negative emotions, beliefs, fears, and patterns that permeate each cell in your body. This cleansing will allow a direct connection to your source and, ultimately, create your freedom.

CHAPTER 2
ALL IS WITHIN

My imaginary boyfriend was Anthony Robbins, the American guru, mentor, and transformation coach. I kept a picture of him in my wallet with the wishful thinking that I could claim him as my own (as did thousands of other women). I had attended many seminars by Anthony Robbins and was in awe of his abilities to transform people's lives, including my own.

Years ago, I attended *Date With Destiny*, my second seminar with Anthony, on the Gold Coast in sunny Queensland, Australia. There were thousands of hyped-up attendees, all eager to see what magic was going to happen in the very large arena. During the group exercises, we were assigned team leaders who supervised us as we completed tasks that reinforced the concepts Anthony had demonstrated. One of the exercises occurred in the evening when the team leaders instructed us to walk along the grassy outdoor area of the venue for our evening session.

We were given a lit candle and, for more than two hours, told to chant the mantra, "All I need is within me now." It was a mesmerising sight, as I viewed the thousands of people following each other, walking over green hills in the moonlight with their flickering candles, repeating the same affirmation. Even though it felt like a spiritual moment, I was unaware the exercise was changing my negative belief systems to something much more powerful.

As I was walking, I asked myself, our time with Anthony Robbins is limited, why have they devoted two hours of the seminar for us to hold a candle and repeat an affirmation I don't know the meaning of? I'd rather be staring into his eyes, shouting for him to pick me when he scanned the room for a volunteer to come on stage.

I was a Mormon at the time and they had taught me the "power" was outside of me and I could find it only in God, Jesus, and the priesthood. I was also suffering from chronic long-term neck pain that kept me struggling in everything I did. The pain was intense, so I regularly visited traditional physical therapists to get relief, but it never lasted.

PAIN IS YOUR INDICATOR TO CHANGE

Shortly after the confusing candlelight mantra, my sister's boyfriend suggested I visit his energy therapist who was "weird and different." I was in extreme pain and desperate to try anything, so I gave it a go despite my misgivings. My upbringing had conditioned me to be fearful of "alternative" therapies and before that, I never ventured outside my comfort zone of chiropractors, massage therapists, doctors, and osteopaths. However, the "norm" was clearly not working and I had nothing to lose. My pain forced me to change and to be more open to other beliefs and opportunities. I have since learned that *pain is an indicator to change.* How much pain do you have to endure before you are willing to change?

The therapist my sister's boyfriend recommended was a kinesiologist, who appeared to be a completely normal guy you would meet on the street. He understood the flow of energy in the body and used biofeedback to read energy fields. In this strange new treatment, the therapist touched various points on my body and tested the strength of certain muscles. When the session was completed, I felt unusually energised. He had connected channels of energy that had been stagnant in my body my entire life.

The second I walked out the door, a little voice in my head said, *this is the path to heal yourself.* This became my introduction to energy healing — the pivotal moment that set me on my life-long mission. I was then to become a proud "weird and different" transforming energy therapist myself, which was the last thing I'd ever imagined as my life's purpose.

In retrospect, the mantra I had repeated, "All I need is within me now," was inferring that I have the power in me to solve any problem in my life. Kinesiology methods are based on the theory that the body will tell you what it needs to heal. After repeating the mantra, the very next day I discovered the therapist who opened up an entirely new and different world of interpreting and understanding energy. If it hadn't been for that opening, I am sure I wouldn't be here today, as I had been so overwhelmed by the emotional and physical pain that followed me everywhere I went.

Now, I am glad to know that I have the power within myself to solve any problem. Everything was divinely orchestrated for me to meet the right person at the right time. The moment I changed my belief system was the moment I regained my ability to guide myself through any challenge that would come my way. I still repeat the mantra and feel guided to solve my own challenges, along with the challenges faced by others who seek my help.

TAKE THE INSANITY PLEA

Since I made the transition from seminar attendee and patient to presenter, I have encountered many women who carry shame, guilt, and blame from childhood. These emotions continue into adulthood, as does the same level of unworthiness that causes them to allow more terrible things to happen to them.

When crazy, incomprehensible things are done to you, you tolerate crazy and incomprehensible behaviour in adulthood. This causes more guilt and negative self-talk, such as, *what the hell was I thinking?* I hear a lot of women say this. Intellectually, they know better, but for reasons that will become clear later, they continue to allow disrespectful or abusive behaviour toward themselves and often toward their children.

As the victim's guilt and shame is compounded, she is stuck, continuing her self-destructive cycle. I openly confess that my past choices have been anything but sane and respectful to myself. There is an entire insane sisterhood who can relate, so you are not alone and I can offer you a plea bargain to get you off the hook. Plead guilty on the grounds of temporary insanity! This will instantly erase guilt for your insane decisions; however, the insanity needs to stop because the plea is only a temporary offer.

When women are taught from an early age that they are unworthy, guilty, or second-class citizens, this compels them to attract and resign themselves to a life of more of the same. A vicious cycle of negative decision-making is put in place. Perhaps you've made decisions in the past that you're not proud of and you'd like to forget. When dealing with these issues, it is useful to find humour in your craziness. Remind yourself you had a moment of "temporary insanity." You didn't know then what you know now. Instead of accumulating even more negative energy, let yourself off the hook!

As Maya Angelou once said, "When you know better, you do better."

TIME TO CHANGE?

Reading this book and going through the healing process is proof that you are attempting to do better, know better, and therefore create better. *"Change"* is the operative word in designing a better life. Change your beliefs, change your choices, change your thoughts, change your emotions, change your friends, change your environment, change your language, change your health, and change your attitude. Are you hearing me, sister? Get used to change. It needs to be a daily occurrence to get fast results without having to endure any more pain.

Leo Tolstoy once said, "Everyone thinks of changing the world, but no one thinks of changing himself." In reality, changing yourself is one of the hardest things to do. Change is difficult because we have a natural instinct to protect ourselves through predictability. When predictability disappears, our sense of security is threatened. The process of change can be even harder for those who have gone through extreme trauma. They often want to maintain the status quo, to feel some sense of control even though the status quo is not serving them. They learnt from past abuse that when things change, they change for the worse. This causes them to react in fear if change is suggested or instigated. Fear is a natural result of conditioning, but it doesn't have to control your life.

Do you find yourself fearing change or fearing the idea of connecting to your feelings? Do you feel panic at the idea of finding hidden secrets or suppressed memories of pain or trauma that lie deep inside you? If you have those feelings, know that you are always protected and your body will only show you what you are capable of dealing with. My favourite saying is, "If you do what you have always done, you will get what you have always got."

I had to be open to alternative healing in order to find my life's calling. I've mentioned before that change is inevitable if you want to alter your outcomes. Prior to being open to change, even though I was longing to be free of my suffering, my mindset was stuck due to decades of experiencing a life of hardship. This left me feeling like a victim, powerless to change anything.

All I knew was that my father destroyed my life and my suffering was the proof. Nobody was holding him accountable for the abuse he inflicted on me, so subconsciously I thought if I got well, then he would be off the hook for the torture I endured.

Now, change has become a daily occurrence. If I don't like the outcomes I am creating, I immediately work out what I need to change to get better outcomes. People who become reacquainted with me say that I seem different. My response is always, "I have changed," and I will continue to do so. I have learnt to embrace change, as I love the opportunity to create something better than before!

Make the commitment and learn to love the idea of change; view it as an exciting challenge and celebrate every change you make. This will give you the freedom of knowing that you have the power within you to create your desired outcomes. *Your life will be your benchmark.*

USE YOUR GPS

I now appreciate the amazing gift of feeling emotionally and physically connected to myself. This connection enhances my intuition, or my personal GPS. When it is nurtured and cultivated, intuition is the most precious tool you will ever possess. It allows you to heal yourself and others. No one gives you a handbook on life (although, some may insist they have one). Even if there was a handbook, it would not be customized to your life, circumstances, and needs. Your personal GPS is entirely yours. It helps you navigate your life unfailingly to achieve your own purpose and greatness.

Whether you are as inexperienced as I was, or whether you are well-versed in the concepts of energy exchange, universal laws, or the law of attraction, you will find a deeper meaning to life and how it operates through the pages of this book. You will understand more completely the mantra, "All I need is within me now," and you can access the power within when you follow the feelings that are continually guiding you.

IT ALL BEGINS WITH ENERGY

The most important habits to form are to think deeply, ask questions, and never take anything for granted. Don't accept that it's normal for things to go wrong and for life to dish up difficult circumstances over which you have no control. Don't accept that physical pain, your computer crashing, or car accidents are random events. I used to think they were, until I began reading energy fields and came to realise that a woman's life is influenced by her own intentions, and by those of the people with whom she associates.

I've experienced the power of other people's energy affecting me in very adverse ways. In my moments of physical pain, financial blocks, accidents, relationship problems, computer malfunctions, and health problems, when I took time to reflect on what was causing them, I would get an impression of a person's face and any negative emotion felt towards me. In the process of removing these negative emotions and connections, I discovered concepts to override the forces against me so that my personal and business life could reach greater heights. The painful mistakes of allowing the wrong people in my life taught me how powerfully others' hidden agendas affected my successes.

Once you understand the universal nature of energy exchange, it will be easier to create the life and relationships you deserve, so read on to find more on how it works.

ENERGY CAN HEAL OR HARM

If people have the power to heal others of life-threatening diseases by using energy, thoughts, prayers, or love, then the opposite can also occur with negative thoughts and intentions. If you analysed your life and took into account the worst things that have happened, there is usually a negative relationship lingering in the background.

Putting two and two together, you could correlate the good and bad things in your life with your relationships. When there are nasty relationships, nasty things happen, which is more apparent when there are bouts of bad luck. I have analysed the results of good and bad relationships to understand how the energy from emotion really works.

One of my experiences related to a work colleague who hid her true feelings. One day, she slipped up and revealed that she sent bucket loads of bad energy to people she didn't like. Back then, I was not conscious enough to realise her agenda towards me was destructive. When she was working in my business, she never voiced any concerns. However, many things started to go wrong when she became dissatisfied.

One incident occurred when she gave me a pat on the back as a sign of affection. An hour later, I experienced excruciating pain in the exact area she had touched. After she resigned, I learnt she was making derogatory comments about me while working in the business.

Negative intentions can cause sharp physical pain. Perhaps this is why betrayal is so often referred to as being "stabbed in the back." In my healings, I have removed "energetic knives" that were the result of others "backstabbing" people with words. When I removed the energetic connection from the "backstabbers," the back pain was removed.

READ THE CLUES

Everyone offers clues about who they really are. If you reflect on your life, you'll see that the most stressful times were usually when someone betrayed you. It can be very painful when you put your trust in a person and he or she takes advantage of you. The outcomes of betrayal are often catastrophic. The person who is not trustworthy is always leaving clues, even if you think they are not. If you didn't see it coming, it means you haven't been taught how to read the signs. You have been taught to give people the benefit of doubt and trust them first. A betrayer will target people who trust easily and don't ask questions. A person who takes from people will target the people who give generously. These types of relationships never last and always cause hurt and anger.

All these interactions leave imprints in your energy field that can linger for years and cause blocks and struggles in your life. If you understand the concept that "energy" comes before a physical creation, then you will understand that your "energy field" is filled with your own thoughts and intentions and all your interactions with — and energy of — people from your past and present.

Einstein said, "Energy is everything" and "Energy cannot be created or destroyed, it can only be changed from one form to another." Learn to read the clues around you to find out if the energy emitted by the people around you is truly positive. I will, through the following chapters, reveal the necessary clues for you to identify.

WHO MAKES THE RULES?

Have you ever felt judged for being different? Have you turned yourself into a Stepford wife, eager to please and playing it safe? Judgements from others can keep people living in fear of being ridiculed or rejected. Society and religion have dictated the rules of how you should look and act. They have provided the unfair criteria of how we should judge others and cause people to feel inferior. Since this archaic thinking is flawed, there is a shift taking place that rejects this conditioning. However, there are still many people who have been conditioned to believe that other people's opinions are more important than their own. This is because they have low self-worth and constantly seek approval to fill an insatiable void within themselves.

It is a constant struggle for a woman to feel okay about caring for herself without being judged as "selfish." Many women feel paralysed trying to be their true selves because being like everyone else feels so much safer. The fear of standing out in a crowd causes them to stay small and hide, even if the result leads to a lonely and unfulfilling life. This programming can be undone. I say openly that I care more about my own feelings than anyone or anything else. I have learned there is no one who is going to consistently care about me, so I have to do it myself. When I genuinely love myself, I have the ability to genuinely love others.

The freedom I have gained from not caring about what others think plays a big part in my success. I give credit to my mother's conditioning. She continually commented, "Who cares what other people think!" Possibly this was her way of feeling better about sending me to school in hand-made purple jumbo corduroy pants, when everyone else was wearing trendy Levi jeans. Her conditioning worked, as I never felt the pressure to conform. All the same, it has taken years of experiencing the negative consequences of caring more about others' needs to now putting my feelings first.

YOUR FEELINGS DO MATTER

I have a new message for all women: *your feelings do matter* and your feelings should be respected and valued. It has become normal for women not to notice the disrespect or second-class position they have been given in life. You will never feel complete unless you learn to unconditionally value and appreciate yourself. When you achieve this level of self-worth you will require others to treat you the same. You are here to "Shine bright like a diamond," as Rihanna's song suggests. Don't settle for anything less and don't accept another person's justification for disrespectful behaviour by saying you owe them, you are too sensitive, or you are over-reacting.

Clarity often comes when we listen to others. One of those moments came for me when my childhood friend said that I should not feel guilty or indebted to my father for helping me financially on the one and only occasion that he did. My friend stated that fathers are supposed to help their children. She proceeded to tell me how wonderful her father was and how he assisted her in so many kind ways as she grew up.

I was left scratching my head, as I had no idea until that moment it was normal for a father to help his child. Worse, it didn't even register in my mind that it was not normal (or even that it was immoral) to emotionally, physically, or sexually abuse a child.

MY MOTHER COMPOUNDED THE PROBLEM

When my father closed the door before abusing us, my mother ignored the screams and pleas for him to stop. She never intervened. I thought my mother loved me, but by allowing his behaviour to continue for years, she was sending a message to me that I was bad, guilty, and deserved to suffer.

All of my beliefs stemmed from my childhood and I could see exactly why my life was so dysfunctional or, to be completely blunt, completely stuffed as an adult. My first long-term relationship was at age thirty-six, when I was first married.

At that point I was still working for British Petroleum. I had progressed in the company and really enjoyed my time there. I was on a nine-year stint, maintaining a good work ethic and making some good friends. I had faithfully served ten years in the Mormon Church by then. However, being a member of the church restricted the pool of available, decent men. The ratio was six women to one man — not very promising odds! I felt I had let the team down as I had failed to marry and reproduce little Mormon people to carry on the legacy of Mormonism, to which I was very committed at the time.

I decided to try online dating in the Mormon community, which led me to meeting my Canadian husband. I'll refer to him as Glen. Dutifully, I kept the law of chastity, which meant no premarital sex (if this rule didn't exist, I know we definitely wouldn't have married!). This restricted the relationship, and truthfully I was more in love with the idea of being married than I was in love with Glen. We married in a Mormon Church stake (a stake is a group of wards/church areas) president's office in Canada, and things didn't improve from there. Glen was a poor communicator, did not know how to have a proper relationship (nor did I for that matter), and read science fiction novels most of his spare time whilst sharing custody of his four children with his ex-wife.

My memories of the entire relationship consist of emotional numbness and enduring physical pain from my whiplash injuries. This often felt so overwhelming that I pondered ways to end my life. The marriage finally ended after three years when I relocated back to Australia.

It was clear I could not maintain healthy relationships and I would have ended the marriage in the first week had I known that I had more choices. Instead, I remained a dutiful and suffering Mormon wife who was under the impression that God was "refining" me through these trials. I didn't know any better and I made bad choices that compounded my suffering.

MY MIND WAS WIRED FOR HARDSHIP

I definitely needed help erasing the corrupted program that ran in my brain 24/7. I came into this life with a pure, clean slate, not knowing anything. My parents wrote words on my blank slate that said my existence was worthy only of abuse. The words and beatings were etched into my soul, and as I grew older, I became the words and beatings, which then became my beliefs. Nothing that anyone told me as an adult could change the sense of ugliness and lowliness that followed me everywhere I went. My father's words and actions could not be erased, no matter how hard I scrubbed my wounded body. All I knew was that life offered struggle and suffering until it became too unbearable to sustain.

Somehow I had to find new memories and words that would heal my soul and re-establish my sense of worth. I had to find a way to delete the corrupted programming that caused this malfunction in my life, and insert a new program that told me I was a precious and deserving woman. Over many decades, I have had a total overhaul and now, I use the most recent "software download" that is defaulted to living a free, deserving, and happy life.

YOUR LIFE REFLECTS YOUR BELIEFS

Even if you aren't dealing with the same corrupted software, I can help you with your new downloads — your new beliefs. We will be going into detail on how to make this happen throughout the chapters of this book. Make a commitment to be kind to yourself, take time out, and take deep breaths when things get uncomfortable. We can finish together in triumph, with passion, and the sense of freedom that you have been longing for. After all, we are all connected and your success is my success.

You have been guided to this book for many reasons. Rest assured that you will be assisted in your process of becoming the person you deserve to be. Your body already knows what is coming up for you. I went through many strange experiences before I confronted my past abuse, and I saw the patterns that would lead up to those moments. I would experience anxiety, fear, overwhelming hurt and betrayal. These physical and emotional patterns manifested weeks prior to my life-changing therapy sessions. When those feelings surfaced again, I began to realise my body was giving me a clue that a huge change was soon to happen. In fact, each time an impactful change was about to take place, chaos preceded it. This pattern still exists today.

PERSIST—IT'S SO WORTH IT!

Even though I wanted to run for the hills before and during my therapy sessions, I forced myself to go through the process, as I knew the truth would set me free. My pain was too much to bear, and the fear of staying the same was greater than the fear of confronting my past. It's like running your first marathon and not giving in when the times get tough. Moving beyond your preconceived limits is exhilarating. It feels so good being on the other side.

CHAPTER 3
SURVIVAL

GATHER THE CLUES

Miss Mather was my grade one teacher, a tall, chubby woman, who let me clean her classroom with a grey feather duster. I took great pride polishing and dusting, while I hummed the song "Sadie (the Cleaning Lady)." It gave me a sense of pride to help a grown-up. The room was small and cramped. We would climb over school desks to get to our places. We all sat closely together on old wooden seats and I remember pinching the smelly, freckled, redheaded boy's bottom next to me. He raised his voice in protest and I would deny I had anything to do with it. Hmm, I wonder if you can accumulate bad karma at the tender age of five?

I invited Miss Mather to my sixth birthday party, and when she arrived, she began chatting with my mother. I looked up and without thinking, I blurted, "Gee, you're so big, Miss Mather." My mum glared at me. I quickly realised how it came across and stammered, "I mean you're so tall ... not fat ... just tall!" It was one of those moments that should've been funny. I mean, really, people? Couldn't everyone just lighten up a little? Apparently not. After Miss Mather left, my mum scolded me for being rude.

My six-year-old voice echoed silently, *you're so stupid! You can never win!* I just wanted approval and love, and no matter what I tried, nothing seemed to work.

My words of self-criticism rang true, as the upcoming year brought the worst possible events. One day I was walking home from school with my classmate, Jeanette Mclean. It was a memory I would spend years trying to erase. Jeanette had a slight lisp, but she spoke with confidence and took delight in playing on my insecurities. She told me that the old derelict house we would pass on our way home was haunted, and warned me that ghosts would come out and scare anyone who walked by.

"They will not!" I protested, hoping she would change her story and say it was an April Fool's joke or that Casper the Friendly Ghost lived there. She didn't reply. Although I put on a brave face, I felt terrified the ghosts would come for me as we walked by. The movie *Ghostbusters* hadn't yet been released; otherwise, I would definitely have known whom to call!

We parted ways at the end of my street. It was an average neighbourhood where nothing out of the ordinary happened. It was an entirely different story inside our house. I would come home from school each day and everything would begin peacefully enough. I would find my mother working in the kitchen, preparing our meal. We were allowed two sweet biscuits for afternoon tea. I was always hungry, so I ate them quickly, hoping our next meal wouldn't be too far away.

The afternoons were uneventful until dinnertime, when my father would arrive home from work. We sat around the laminated dinner table, with my father at the head. We ate quietly, hoping we would make it through without him hitting one of us.

Whenever he slapped us over the head, he would yell, "I'll knock your bloody brains out!" It didn't make sense, especially, when he called me stupid. I would fester inside and blame him, as he hit me so many times over the head it was a wonder I had any brains left.

My brother swallowed his pea's whole, as he detested the taste. My younger sister sat placidly, dutifully eating all her food. When we finished, we were required to ask permission to leave the table, and it was always a relief when we could. It was like being in a class you hated, with your least favourite teacher, waiting for the bell to go so you could run outside for recess.

Even at that young age I saw my father as the enemy, so I constantly tried to avoid him. Intense hatred and resentment filled my heart. He controlled us with intimidation, but I wasn't going to succumb, even at six years of age! He knew how I felt, and he was going to find ways to punish me until I relented. It was too bad I didn't fake it, as it would have saved me from quite a few beatings, but sucking up to my father's intimidation just wasn't an ability that "God" bestowed upon me.

Our bedtime was around 7.30 p.m. Out of fear, we brushed our teeth religiously. My father would apply toothpaste to our toothbrushes so he could monitor our obedience of our brushing routine. We didn't want to be caught out or we would pay with a beating from the belt. He kept his thick, green, canvas army belt hanging on the back of the kitchen door. Every time we opened the door, its large gold buckle would smash against the door, to remind us of the threat of punishment. My father acted more like a power-mad drill sergeant than a loving caregiver. I wondered if I drew the short straw when God was assigning us parents whom he then commanded us to honour and obey.

THE GHOST STORY

My sister was eighteen months younger than I, so she was around five years old when we shared the back bedroom. Above my bed hung an angel plaque with the inscription *Guardian Angel Watch Over Me Tonight*. My headboard had a Road Runner sticker, and my sister's had Porky Pig, which I teased her about. I had a right, as the Road Runner was much faster than a stuttering, fat, pink pig!

That night, after being sent to bed, Jeanette's ghost warning began to fill my mind. My growing feeling of dread brought on an anxiety attack. I asked my sister if I could jump into her bed, as I was too scared to sleep alone. As expected, she agreed, as she liked to keep the peace. I climbed into her bed feeling some relief, but it was short-lived.

A few minutes later, my father walked by the bedroom — it seemed strange that he checked on us. He was usually consumed with his favourite TV programmes so we tended to have little communication with him, especially after our bedtime. But that night, he had his radar on red alert. He was looking to catch me for something that would give him reason to unleash the rage that he could not contain.

"Get into your own bed!" he shouted. I quickly jumped out of Donna's bed and into my own. I lay quietly and tried to sleep, until the fear of ghosts coming to get me returned. I crept back into my sister's bed, praying to God my father wouldn't return. I was wrong, as he caught me out of my own bed for the second time.

Without a word, he walked back into the kitchen and took the army belt off the door. I knew I was a goner. I was shaking before he even closed the bedroom door behind him. He grabbed my skinny arm and yanked me out of bed, so he could swing the belt with full force.

Tears rolled down my face, as I knew what was coming. I tried to place both my hands behind my back as he pulled down my pyjama pants. He lifted the belt high in the air.

"This will teach you to disobey me. Don't you ever do that again!" He swung his arm back to get as much force as possible. The belt hit my bare bottom with a snap. Terrible pain followed.

Again and again, he swung, until his anger and rage finally subsided. I was a mess of tears and hurt. I climbed back into my bed with my traumatised body. *Big Brother, can somebody please call 911 and remove the psycho drill sergeant from the house, so I don't have to add another decade of expensive therapy to my already screwed-up life?*

Long after he was gone, I lay in bed, wide-awake and terrified. I was still fearful of the ghosts. At 5.00 a.m., I heard a dragging noise outside the bedroom window. It was on the driveway, coming closer. Fear took control, as I imagined ghosts had plotted my death and were coming for me. I was too scared to get out of bed, yet simultaneously too scared to stay in my bed. The dragging noise kept getting louder. It was not my imagination; the ghosts were definitely coming towards our window! My fear became overwhelming and I couldn't contain it. I screamed bloody murder, and everyone ran into the room. My mum, dad, brother, and sister were all staring at me, not knowing why I was screaming.

As I calmed down, in between sobs, I told them about Jeanette, and the ghosts coming to get me. I explained that I heard them coming up the driveway. My mother responded that ghosts were not real and told me that Jeanette made up the story. My brother clarified that his slippers had made the noise outside. He had walked to the front of the house to collect the milk bottles and was returning along the driveway directly outside our window. Not long after the explanation, everyone went back to bed, satisfied I was not being murdered. I lay in my bed, still in shock and feeling numb.

At 7.30 a.m., exhausted, I crawled out of bed and made my way to the kitchen. No one mentioned anything as I ate my two Weetabix with milk before leaving for school. When I walked home with Jeanette, I challenged her.

"You just made up those ghost stories, didn't you?"

She admitted she did. We parted ways and head down, dragging my feet along Gilmore Road, I reluctantly returned home. My hell on Earth.

Soon after, the torturous sexual abuse from my father began. Earth calling God, Earth calling God, bring back humanity. **PLEASE?**

SURVIVAL MECHANISMS

Disconnecting from my thoughts, feelings, and memories was essential to get through my childhood. This left me feeling frozen and unhappy as I reached adulthood. My life was a pantomime of what I thought normal should look like. I had no concept of how it felt to be secure, loved, or happy. I simply buried my feelings and tried to live a life based on the images I'd seen and books I read.

Not everyone experiences the extremes of physical and sexual abuse, but scars from childhood are damaging, regardless of whether you faced neglect, abuse, divorce, the death of a parent or sibling, or instability of any kind. All of these experiences imprint on your soul, or energy field, and continue to manifest in your adult life until you've acknowledged them and healed the pain they caused.

At twenty three years of age, I moved to Italy to escape my family and the painful memories. I had spent my teens getting into deep trouble: smoking, drinking, consuming drugs, and allowing myself to be used by men. I didn't value my mind or my body. This often brought me to my knees, praying to God to end my life or find some sort of relief. After a couple of years living in Florence, I was intuitively guided to join the Mormon Church, which ultimately changed my destiny.

Spending a part of my life in the church was a significant turning point for me. At the time, it offered the support system I was lacking. It propelled me to relinquish the self-destructive behaviours I'd undertaken to fill the emptiness in my life. For this reason, I am grateful to church members for showing me a different way to live. My years of church service prepared my mind and body for the journey that led me to heal myself. As a faithful member, I had to forgo all vices, such as alcohol, smoking, tea, coffee, and other addictive substances and behaviours. This cleared my physical system, and paved the way for future healing. I was finally on my way!

After I had joined the church the crying episodes began. My body was getting ready to release the emotions stored in it.

FLASHBACKS

My childhood memories were very vague. I continually experienced emotions of anger and unworthiness. There was a lingering unanswered question as to why I felt so bad. It was like a poison running through my veins that I could not expunge. The question that persisted was, "What use is it to experience so much deep and overwhelming pain when I would rather be dead?"

One of my questions was answered when a sudden recollection of my childhood came to mind. While I was kneeling beside my bed, reciting my daily prayers, I was not thinking of anything particular or different from any other time when a distinct memory flashed before me. As I stood up to make my way to the kitchen, a vision of my six-year-old self stopped me in my tracks. I was standing on the cold bathroom floor, wondering why I was suffering from so much pain. I remembered thinking, *what the hell just happened to me? Why do I feel violated and uncomfortable?*

A flash of insight revealed that it was the morning after my father sexually abused me. I was enraged to realise as an adult what my father had done to me. The image was not new. It had always existed, shut away, waiting to reveal itself when I had the strength to face the truth of what happened. This revelation was setting me free; however, not knowing what to do or how to respond sent me spiralling downward all over again.

DENIAL: THE BEST DEFENCE?

When a woman informs her family that she experienced sexual abuse, it's sometimes the case she will be met with denial and face accusations that she made it up. When others deny abuse or even blame the victim, it can feel so painful that many survivors won't confront the abuser, much less tell anyone else what happened. Survivors can live silently with their horror and pain until it eats away at them, and their body can no longer contain the emotions. I have no doubt my chronic pain was untreatable for so many years because it was a build-up of toxic energy from burying this secret.

My father was charming in public; however, he was a different person behind closed doors. He belittled my mother daily, eventually leaving her for another woman. He claimed he owned everything, as he had paid for everything with his money. Even my school reports (as bad as they were) he claimed were his, as he paid for my education. It's similar to the Bible, where the best known scriptures preach love and compassion, while lesser known ones encourage discrimination, abuse, slavery, war, sacrifice, and intolerance. People are conditioned to live the same way, hide the acts of abuse and intolerance, and outwardly live as law-abiding citizens.

My mother completed a double degree in psychology after her divorce from my father. She claimed her reasoning was to understand why we became such a dysfunctional family. I was the one who really went off the tracks. I phoned her straight after my flashback and described what I remembered, thinking she would be supportive, hoping she would offer some kind of explanation or apology for the hell we endured under their roof.

To my surprise, my mother denied my father would ever do such a terrible thing. She said he always deplored paedophiles, saying they deserved to be punished. My mother, to this day, has no idea of the struggle I went through. She still complains that at age fourteen I "turned crazy" and became an uncontrollable, angry teenager for no reason. It just goes to show that people measure another's life by comparing it to their own. I was self-destructive and ran away from home, smoked from an early age, and got caught up in other addictive behaviours, just searching for a way out of my emotional hell, and my mother can't understand why. I'm still wondering what they taught during her psychology classes, as I seem to be a complete enigma to her. I know I'm a classic textbook case of what happens to abused children. If I shared all the stories I've heard from women who endured similar struggles as my own, this book would become a never-ending series.

So many years later, my mother still protests, "I just don't know what happened; you were such a good child. You were my little helper, always at my side." She continues to defend her position as a mother and says it was my own fault that I turned out the way I did. She's still angry with me for losing the plot and putting her through unnecessary stress.

This denial has left me with very few family connections. Their silence, denial, and minimising my abuse only perpetuated my pain. The last time I spoke with my father was when I confronted him about the sexual abuse he perpetrated on me. His reply was not to deny what he had done, but to say I was making potentially dangerous accusations against him. He then contacted my mother, to whom he'd stopped speaking, and diagnosed me as — and I quote — "psychologically disturbed."

Where was Judge Judy when I needed her? She could have sorted this crap out in seconds. I don't suppose she would have done house calls back then...?

The process of healing my life has been gut wrenching, and much harder because nobody wanted to address the elephant in the room. I had to find the truth in order to be set free. Over the years I have met and worked with women who are dealing with denial and blame, and I can relate to all of them. Denial comes in many forms, and even the women themselves often refute what happened to them or the significance of the impact of abuse. Denial is a coping mechanism, because the truth that the people who are supposed to love and protect you have abused you is often too painful to confront.

Moving on from your past takes more than positive thinking, more than talking about what happened, and much more than attending workshops or seminars. You need to reconnect to your own energy source, or spirit, for any of those things to take effect. When you are trying to reach out and find the courage to tell the truth, if the abuse is denied it feels like it is reinforced. In essence, the denial says you are a liar, your pain is not valid, and your feelings don't matter. It can be more difficult to heal from emotional or physical pain and move on when no one will admit any wrongdoing, or take responsibility.

Don't be discouraged if others have denied your experience, or if you fear you can't recover your self-worth. This book will offer the words that should have been spoken to validate your experience. The exercise at the end of this chapter will start the process of discovering the events and people that have had a negative impact on your life.

SIGNS OF DISCONNECTION

The feeling of being disconnected can come from past abuse, or from other traumas related to divorce, abandonment, or not having a supportive network. The following list highlights the signs, symptoms, and dysfunctional behaviours that can reflect a disconnection or a shutting down of emotions. See which ones you can relate to.

1) ANXIETY:

The Mayo Clinic, in the USA, reports that victims of abuse are most likely to be diagnosed with anxiety disorders. Anxiety can cause nightmares, severe panic attacks, and extreme fears that inhibit socialising. When survivors encounter situations that remind them of their past, they often experience physical conditions such as chest tightening, excessive sweating or hyperventilation. Fear of sexual intimacy is a common result of sexual abuse and can lead to feeling overwhelmed, without understanding why.

2) ANGER:

It is a normal reaction for survivors to feel anger toward their circumstances, the abusers, and the people who did not protect them. Anger can also be directed within, particularly when the victim believes that he or she should have stopped the abuse. Those who suppress their anger can experience depression, illnesses, or reach a boiling point, during which they feel they are going crazy, and want to explode. Expressing anger is a necessary process for victims to heal. It can be managed in a constructive manner to facilitate healing.

3) DISSOCIATION:

This is a feeling of being disconnected from people and life. It can manifest as feeling emotionless, numb, confused, and having out-of-body experiences. This feeling can occur during or after abuse, to help the victim avoid the associated pain. Memories of abuse can be deeply repressed and the victim can unconsciously choose distractions to avoid dealing with them.

4) POST-TRAUMATIC STRESS DISORDER:

PTSD is usually associated with war veterans who encounter trauma in battle, and their body exhibits shock symptoms. Research also shows that PTSD is prevalent among people who have experienced any traumatic event, including violence, physical abuse, civil unrest, natural disasters, or major accidents. Symptoms can manifest as nightmares, flashbacks, anxiety, fear, rage, and crying outbursts.

5) SHAME:

Victims feel guilt and shame when they believe they deserved the abuse, were responsible for it, or could have stopped it. Those who groom a child for abuse manipulate and condition the child to think that he or she deserves it.

6) SELF-DESTRUCTIVE BEHAVIOUR:

Often survivors self-medicate with drugs, alcohol, or engage in self-harm, such as burning or cutting themselves. When there is ongoing abuse, victims neglect their health, sabotage their own success, or seek out scenarios where abuse is repeated.

7) Trust Issues:

In abuse or trauma, the victims learn they can't trust others to keep them safe. In adulthood this manifests as being over-controlling and overbearing. Fear of intimacy is common for women, as they feel vulnerable in intimate relationships.

8) Physical Symptoms:

When emotions are suppressed, the body shuts down the energy flow in the meridians (acupressure lines through the body) and physical symptoms appear. The conditions will manifest initially in the weakest areas of the body, resulting in issues such as skin conditions, headaches, migraines, constipation, high blood pressure, low immune system, dizziness, tiredness, tight jaw, and neck disorders. They can also trigger genetic disorders and other health problems.

THE PATH TO RECONNECT YOURSELF

Reconnecting to your feelings is the first step to healing. If you don't feel connected, you aren't truly present or aware of yourself, your surroundings, or other people — and your body cannot receive the healing needed. You stay frozen in time, trying to keep your world safe from any more abuse or neglect. You operate in survival mode, and nothing can penetrate your barriers in order to help you. You become your own worst enemy.

Eventually, I became aware I had built walls that kept me in my own emotional prison. I tried many methods to break them down and eventually they fell away. This created a better canvas for my healing to begin. With any journey, you need a clear road to travel. Roadblocks, potholes, debris, and diversions must be removed, so you can easily and joyfully arrive at your destination.

Move along, move along, we're coming through, people!

WERE YOU NEGLECTED OR ABUSED?

Childhood trauma can result from any negative behaviour, even if a parent had good intentions. When a parent spends time away from his or her child, working or engaging in other activities without first meeting the child's needs, the child may feel rejected. If the parent neglects to reassure and provide sufficient love and encouragement, the child will develop feelings of unworthiness and abandonment. This will have lasting negative consequences.

Some people cannot recall their childhood memories. This can indicate their childhood was unhappy, so they became disconnected and emotionally absent. When this occurs with my clients, I ask specific questions to reach memories they find difficult to recall, such as home and school memories. It's a form of detective work: the more a person describes her past, the more quickly the memories return. Another helpful approach is to compare people's upbringing to their children's. I question if the same experiences they encountered would affect their own children.

This questioning process allows for reflection on upbringing from a parent's perspective and, for the first time, it can bring awareness to the hurt and neglect experienced in childhood. It seems easier for people to connect with others' pain than their own.

ASKING FOR ASSISTANCE

The Forensic Healing Protocol assists with uncovering the right information. Before I begin any healing session, I use the Forensic Healing Protocol, which contains "Opening the Case" statements. This includes making requests to invoke enlightened beings, divine guidance, divine protection, and divine blessings to be present. I request that I become a pure, clear conduit, and connection for the healing to occur. Starting this way sets the intention to attract the right energy to safely reveal the information needed. It has never failed, as many clients and students have their memories restored, and I can receive information intuitively. As a practitioner, I am often the first person to hear a victim's lifelong secrets. I think if every abused woman on the planet were to release her pain, the tears would fill an ocean.

To begin moving forward in life, it is important to be aware of what happened in your past. Many people are unaware how their childhood has affected them. A child's core emotional needs are love, stability, safety, and encouragement. When these are absent, a child will find ways to blame himself or herself, which creates lifelong negative beliefs and patterns.

FREEING WOMEN EXERCISE
KNOWING YOURSELF

As parts of my childhood memories returned, I tried to make sense of it all. There were many pieces of the puzzle that started to come together as I retraced my steps. It started to make sense of why I experienced high levels of anxiety and panic attacks, felt unsafe, and wanted to lock my bedroom door at night when my father visited my home.

As you start working through the exercises in this chapter, you too will have this experience of seeing the parts of the jigsaw puzzle of your life gradually coming together. This is the first step towards reconnecting with yourself and building a strong connection to your internal GPS.

STEP 1: THE HURT LETTER HEALING

Find a fresh notebook for the following writing exercises and give it a title such as: *My Journey to Free Myself*. This will be your journal as you move through this book to find and heal yourself. Use it as a guide to chart your progress.

Begin by writing yourself a letter about the painful times in your childhood and how they affected you. This is a suggested structure for your letter;

1. Recall the times from your childhood where you have felt suppressed, alone, abandoned, bullied, hurt, judged, unappreciated or violated.
2. Describe the above feelings and put them into words.
3. Write as if you were the observer of those life events.

Here's an example:

Dear Marisa,

When you were young, you felt abused and hurt by your father. Every time he beat you with the belt, it stung. It hurt when he hit you, or pulled your ears so hard they bled. You lived in so much fear of his criticism, calling you stupid, idiot, black sheep, ugly, and a whore.

He favoured your sister and would point her out and say, "Isn't she beautiful?" You stood beside her as if it was normal to be treated as a second-class citizen. You learned to hate him with a passion, as he spent years trying to control you. You never hated someone for as long as your father.

You felt unworthy, like a helpless victim, as your mother didn't protect you or stand up for herself. Your older brother was taught to disrespect you. He savoured the times he could get you into trouble so your beatings would increase. Life was a struggle, and you knew no other way. The sexual abuse changed who you were, and changed your connections with everyone, especially men. It taught you to feel unworthy of love and respect. It filled you with so much darkness and physical and emotional pain that you wanted to end your life.

It was awful seeing you cry for hours in your bedroom. After beating you, your father would walk in and gloat as you cried. It was just too much for such a little person to endure. I saw you thinking that God was punishing you because you were sinful and bad. There just didn't seem to be a way to heal your broken and tortured soul.

It taught you to allow others to take advantage of you and for you to give without ever receiving. There were times when you felt hunted down by your father, as he grabbed you off the street by your hair and threw you in the car like you were a wild animal. Life was sucked out of you and you felt like dirt on the ground.

Some of the schoolteachers were no better. In grade two, you watched a nun humiliate a poor little boy, by grabbing him and pulling down his pants to cane him on his bare bottom in front of the class. Many years later, you saw him receiving food from the Salvation Army shelter, wondering how much damage the nun had done to an already abused boy. All of these things caused you to stop feeling, and fuelled your depression. It's a wonder you ever survived, and not surprising you spent decades wanting to end your life.

STEP 2: FIND THE CLUES

Engage in some detective work and ask people from your childhood for their memories of your upbringing. Specifically, ask them what they recall of your family relationships and your behaviour. Speak to school friends, extended family — anyone from your past. Scan your family photos, school reports, and references, anything that reminds you of your past, and look for clues. In one of my primary school reports, the teacher mentioned I was a daydreamer and emotionally absent. When I started to read my reports, feelings of sadness surfaced, and I started to realise the amount of neglect I endured. As hard as that was, I started to see more clearly, and gained a deeper understanding of myself.

This process may cause you to feel as if you are moving blindly through a dark tunnel, searching for safety. However, your strength and determination *will* help you find the light at the end of the tunnel! You will find a bright shining sun offering warmth, safety, and comfort.

FLASHBACKS AND REVISITING MY HOME

When I had the bathroom flashback of the morning after my father abused me, something urged me to visit my childhood home. I wanted to know if I could learn more about what had happened. I followed my instincts and drove to the house. I sat in my car, looking at the untidy and dishevelled house I had lived in twenty years earlier. It was much neater when I lived there. It felt strange, as all the surrounding houses had been well maintained and neat, and my old house looked like it didn't belong. I took a deep breath, and slowly walked up to the front door. My heart raced as the urge to run back to my car overtook me. I experienced fear and anxiety as if I were still living there. But I didn't run. I knew I had to go ahead with my plans, even though I wasn't prepared for what I was going to say.

Timidly, I knocked at the door and a polite lady opened it and greeted me. I told her that I had lived in her house many years ago, and was hoping she would let me enter as I was trying to recollect what happened to me as a child. As soon as I completed the last sentence, I burst into tears. She saw my distress and invited me in while I wiped my face. There was barely any communication between us as I walked from the hall to the kitchen, then to the bedroom where the abuse happened. The house looked much smaller than I remembered. The rooms were dark even though it was the middle of a spring day. The owner had pulled down all the blinds. I spent a few minutes inside the house, thanked her, and quickly left. My heart was racing the entire time. I'm sure it was strange for her, too — to have a crying woman she'd never met wanting to view her house.

I knew the moment I spoke to the owner that my feelings were validated. My body has proven it to me over and over again: it knows better than I do and reacts when it confirms truth. As I have gathered the clues, I've come to know the truth about many things, and the process has set me free.

CHAPTER 4
ADMISSION

ANGER-A MANIFESTATION OF PAIN

The moment I relayed to old family friends that my father had sexually abused me, I realised how much anger was stored in my body. After chatting casually at the dining room table, the conversation suddenly became more serious. I had a close relationship with these people because they understood some of the weird family dynamics that went on and often sympathised with me. I divulged what my father had done to me. My mother, who was in the adjacent room, overheard my comments. She immediately came in and defended my father, saying she did not believe he would be capable of doing such a thing.

The moment I heard her words, a wave of anger overtook my entire being. I slammed my fist on the kitchen table so hard that I thought I broke my wrist. I screamed that in no uncertain terms was she to f***ing repeat those words again. I yelled and questioned why she would believe the biggest lying A-hole on the planet, over *me*. I never wanted to hear my mother defend my father again.

It felt surreal and, for the first time in my life, I knew I had no control over my rage or what I might do. I had to restrain myself from breaking everything in sight. In that split second, I thought I was capable of murder. Luckily for everyone present, there were no weapons close at hand.

The experience made me realise that I was angry not only with my father, but also with my mother for not protecting me, and for choosing to live in denial. She would not accept the truth — that she married a man who molested their daughter — as that would classify her as a bad mother and damage her image. It was the same pattern when I ran away from home. My whole family ended up in court, in front of a juvenile judge who knew I ran away because of my father's physical abuse. The judge gave me a choice of going to a foster home or returning home with my parents. I was in a deep depression and responded that I didn't care what happened, so I was sent back home. My mother instructed all of us to keep everything that had happened, *a secret.*

Acknowledging the truth would mean too much guilt for my mother to bear. Existing in denial was her way of being able to live each day thinking that her children were raised with adequate food, clothing, and the tolerable amount of abuse and punishment that society permitted for her time.

- Secrets are the opposite of Truth
- Secrets bind you to your Pain
- Denial blinds you to your Betrayer
- The Truth sets you Free
- Choose to be Free

RELEASING THE ANGER

Anger is a normal emotion that can range from mild annoyance to intense rage. It is a feeling that is accompanied by biological changes in your body. When you get angry, your heart rate and blood pressure rise and stress hormones are released. This can cause you to shake, become hot and sweaty, and feel out of control. Anger is associated with feeling hurt, frightened, disappointed, worried, embarrassed, or frustrated. Suppressed anger has been implicated in serious illnesses, especially heart disease. It takes a lot of energy to maintain anger, so it will deplete your energy and motivation.

The idea of expressing anger can be frightening. This is because you connect anger with the person who inflicted pain, trauma, or control over you. Your perpetrator expressed anger through control and did not give you permission to express your hurt. Years of constantly suppressing your emotions can build up to the point you feel you have a volcano of emotions inside. This creates a fear the volcano could erupt if you connect with your suppressed anger. The normal and natural process of grieving from hurt, suffering, and pain comes in five stages. These stages are necessary for a person to feel whole and move on from the past.

THE FIVE STAGES OF HEALING

STAGE 1: Denial, numbness, and shock are all fight-or-flight responses. Blocking the reality of what you've been through gives you time and space to deal with what happened later. This stage serves to protect you from experiencing the intensity of the pain in your heart.

STAGE 2: Rationalising may involve thoughts to justify what happened or to make sense of the situation. You may become preoccupied thinking how things could have been different or how you could have responded differently. If this stage is not resolved, intense feelings of remorse or guilt may interfere with the healing process.

STAGE 3: Depression. This stage occurs after you realise the true extent of your pain and experience feelings of injustice and helplessness. It may cause sleep and appetite problems, low energy, poor concentration, and crying spells. A person may feel loneliness, emptiness, isolation, and self-pity.

STAGE 4: Anger. This reaction occurs when you try to move on from the feelings of helplessness and injustice. It is acknowledging the hurt as you struggle to move forward. You may feel anger at God and/or towards life in general.

STAGE 5: Acceptance. This is the last process needed for healing. It involves coming to terms with your pain. It is the final acknowledgment of the ugly truth of what occurred in your past so you can accept it and take the steps to move on.

FREEING WOMEN EXERCISE:
EXPRESS AND FEEL

It takes strength and courage to express and communicate your pain to the people who hurt you. It can expose your vulnerable side, the very part that you want to protect and keep safe. When you communicate your emotions, you move out of your comfort zone. This can be an opportunity for growth and healing as long as your feelings are acknowledged and respected.

There are always risks that you take when confronting the person who hurt you. As you will read further in this chapter, I took a risk and it remains today one of my worst adult memories. Therefore, please be reassured that this exercise can be done without having to confront the person who hurt you. It is a role-playing exercise that can achieve a similar outcome.

Remind yourself you are safe to feel and connect. Allow yourself to finally express every traumatic emotion that your inner child was feeling. This is the time to let loose and use profanity to your heart's content. You need to feel the pain and let it all out for the other person to hear *as if they were present.* Make a commitment to finally say what you felt and what you would have said if you were defending a little child who was hurt by your perpetrator.

This is the moment to be completely truthful. You have been preparing to finally stand up for yourself. It can take time for you to access these hidden emotions. To help you retrieve them, you can start with the pain and suffering you feel right now. Focus on these feelings and trace them back. *The source is your childhood pain.* Realise how the offender from your past has infiltrated so many areas of your life and how important it is to hold them accountable for their actions. This exercise can be done alone or with a friend who acts as the person who hurt you. Your friend can hold the pillow for you to hit and punch out your anger and hurt.

STEP 3: THE EMOTIONAL RELEASE

1. Identify the person in your childhood who has hurt you. Rate your anger or hurt out of ten (ten is the highest score).
2. Find a place where you will feel comfortable to shout, scream, cry, or swear.
3. Use a pillow to hit and punch. Place it on a couch or bed.
4. Imagine the pillow is the person who hurt you.
5. Read your "Hurt Letter" then express everything you are feeling while hitting and punching the pillow.

You might shout statements like:

- "I hate you for torturing me and forcing me do things I didn't want to do."
- "I feel judged and guilty for all the times you criticised what I did."
- "I have no worth because you are a perverted f***ing sleazeball who molested me."
- "I hate who you are and what you have done to me."

And so on.

When you have completely vented, let yourself cry until you feel you have released the toxic emotions inside you. Allow yourself time and space to feel, release, and receive comfort. This process can be draining, and you may feel as if you have gone through the wringer. This is completely normal. You may also experience tingling and energy pulsing through your body. This is because energy will naturally start moving through channels and meridians in your body that have been blocked and stagnant.

THE WOMAN THAT WAS NEVER ANGRY

I've heard many times the phrase, "I'm not angry, I am just hurt and disappointed." However, if the person making those statements were really honest with herself, she would find the natural outcome of feeling hurt is anger. I have also encountered the opposite with some clients. One woman came to see me about her husband, who had an affair after thirty years of what seemed a good marriage. She continued to explain that he left her for a younger and prettier woman. Strangely, the woman then told me she wasn't angry with him or the new girlfriend, which I confirmed energetically. There was no anger present in her energy field.

The woman showed me a picture of her face two weeks after she learned of the affair. I could not recognise her face in the photo, as it was distorted. There was no resemblance to the woman who was sitting opposite me, showing me this picture. It was more like the elephant man than her real face. The client had suppressed her anger to the extent that it dissolved in her body and manifested in her face. In Chinese medicine, the emotion of anger is connected to the liver and gallbladder, and the liver is responsible for skin conditions.

I surmised that she "ate" her anger. She confirmed my suspicions and explained that when she was a child she was taught to never be angry, as anger was wrong and sinful. She was taught to turn the other cheek, forgive everyone, and not harbour bad feelings.

THE APOLOGY STORY

From age thirty, I realised my mind and body were in utter chaos. I struggled to find a way to heal and move forward. I was a ball of raw emotion and just followed my instincts on what to do, even though I was not really conscious of my thought patterns.

A few months after the memories of sexual abuse surfaced, I initiated contact with my father. I had already spoken to him a few years prior about the physical abuse, which he brushed aside and blamed everyone but himself. Then, I chose to write him a letter and told him I knew he had sexually abused me as a child and I wanted an apology. I waited for a reply but nothing was forthcoming.

Six months later I was invited to meet with him at his house whilst I was on holidays visiting my sister, who lived in his state. My father advised my sister he would speak with me in response to my letter. I was still naive and yearning for some sort of justice or apology so I could move on in my life. I agreed to meet with him in the hope he would say sorry and I could feel better about myself and release my pain, guilt, and shame. After all, he was inviting me to talk to him. What other reason could there be?

My father made plans with my sister that she would drive me to his house so we could meet. As soon as I was dropped off, my sister and my father's girlfriend left the house. I then realised I was inside his "territory," which gave him an unfair advantage. That I would be alone felt contrived and I suddenly realised I had stepped into a trap.

I had no way out of the area where he lived. I was unfamiliar with the neighbourhood and did not know my sister's address, or how to get back there. Mobile phones were not common at that time so there was no easy way for me to call her. Before my sister left, we set a time for her return. She said they would go for a coffee and come back on time to pick me up.

My heart was racing as my father told me to sit down at the kitchen table. I could sense he wasn't happy to see me. He had a very angry demeanour so, out of fear, I obediently sat down.

"You want an apology?" he said, removing a letter from his shirt pocket and handing it to me. "Here it is."

Anxiously I began scanning each line of the full-page typed letter.

…I am sorry you were ever born.
I am sorry you were a whore for a daughter.
I am sorry you joined a religious cult…

The entire page was a list of reasons he was sorry I was in his life.

I can't remember the entire letter, as I crunched it up and threw it down on his kitchen table. He had obviously spent a lot of time documenting my life of disappointments and fabricating details to justify his abuse. There was no denial of any of the things he had done to me, just reasons why I should never have been born, and inferences that I deserved all of the abuse and more. I know he didn't count on his secret getting out after so many years. He was in attack mode, trying to take away my power, and accuse me of being insane. I felt shocked and detached.

My father laughed when he saw the distress on my face. I panicked and tried to leave his house but I couldn't open the screen door. My father laughed even more. My stress level increased as I tried a different door. I felt trapped the same way I'd been as a child. I eventually unlocked the wire screen door while my father continued his sarcastic laugh. I wanted to run as far away as possible. But I couldn't — I had no phone, no transport, no money, and no address for my sister's house. My only option was to run and wait nearby.

Feeling isolated and overwhelmed, I stood in the middle of an adjacent empty block of land. Time dragged and I felt like screaming for help. The insects were terrible, and the wait was one of the worst in my life. My sister, in her regular tardy manner, eventually came back — an hour late. Her excuse was that my father's girlfriend deliberately stretched out the time, insisting on returning later than agreed. My heart felt as if it had been stabbed with a knife and twisted. This was not what I had imagined, expected, or planned.

Reflecting now, I should have known better. My father had never apologised for anything; his nature is to blame everyone but himself. He tried to instil guilt and beat me into submission. Why the hell had I thought anything might change? This was my wake up call, and the final straw of our relationship. I have not spoken to him since.

THE POWER OF APOLOGY

The devastation of not receiving an apology allowed me to fully understand the significance and power of receiving one. An apology releases the guilt and shame from the hurt person. When the wrongdoer apologises, he or she is saying to the other person: you did not deserve to be treated the way you were treated, and you are not guilty of any wrongdoing. *The apology lifts the weight of the world off someone's shoulders.*

Research shows that receiving an apology has a noticeable, positive, physical effect on the body. An apology affects the body systems of the person receiving it — blood pressure decreases, heart rate slows, and breathing becomes steadier.

An apology helps the receiver heal and forgive the wrongdoer. Even though it might seem justified to retain anger towards another person for wrong actions, harbouring anger and refusing forgiveness is harmful for the person who holds onto these emotions.

Nelson Mandela once said, "Resentment is like drinking poison and then hoping it will kill your enemies." Negative emotions can eat away at your insides and leave you feeling unwell. Finding ways to move on and let go of anger and hurt is paramount to achieving health and happiness. *Receiving an apology is the most powerful and fastest way to achieving this.*

An apology from the wrongdoer is not easy to ask for, and when you are refused one, it can feel like salt being rubbed into an open wound. When the wrongdoer will not say that he or she is sorry, it causes a second injury to the hurt person. In essence the wrongdoer is saying to the victim that the abuse and neglect was deserved. This enforces emotions of guilt and shame. Even as an adult, you may intellectually know you did not deserve hurtful treatment in childhood, however, your foundation is built on your childhood. If your "inner child" still feels guilty and hurt, this can keep you stuck and struggling to move on. Your foundation overrides your adult intellect and affects your relationships, decisions, and self-worth. *A sincere apology can help to rebuild this foundation.*

FREEING WOMEN EXERCISE:

THE APOLOGY METHOD

Often when I am treating a client who harbours anger towards an ex-spouse, partner, or family member, I am able to search in her childhood and find another unresolved hurt. The client may have a raging anger that rates 10/10 in her present life; however when the hurt from her childhood is resolved, the anger she directs towards others diminishes.

There are three meaningful steps to achieve a powerful apology that removes blame and restores dignity and self-worth. Whilst you can't undo the past, you can repair the harm that was done to you. In the following exercise, you are going to offer your hurt inner child an apology.

A powerful and meaningful apology includes the following three phases:

1. Acknowledgment of the Hurt

The wrongdoer should show sincerity and acknowledge in detail the specific things he said or did that were wrong. This conveys that the wrongdoer understands the level of hurt that took place. It shows more sincerity by being specific instead of minimising actions; he takes responsibility for hurting the other person.

2. Remove the Guilt and Blame

By articulating to the hurt person that she is not guilty or at fault, the burden and guilt she has been carrying are relieved. The wrongdoer returns the blame and responsibility to himself /herself and ceases to make excuses for his/her actions.

3. Restitution: What Should Have Occurred

To help the hurt person recover from the damage, the wrongdoer communicates what should have occurred instead. The wrongdoer repairs the damage as they describe with words of compassion and love, the different responses and actions that should have taken place. The wrongdoer describes to the hurt person that he or she should have been protected, nurtured, and loved. He or she should have felt safe, valued, and acknowledged. This has the effect of erasing the pain and hurt of the past, and replacing it with a loving foundation.

FREEING WOMEN EXERCISE:
THE APOLOGY

STEP 4: RATE YOUR ANGER

Begin rating your anger towards the person who has hurt you the most, on a scale of one to ten — ten being the most intense anger, zero being none.

Begin writing your inner child an apology letter using the three phases outlined above. Refer to your "Hurt Letter" in Chapter 3, which details the hurtful experiences from childhood.

Respond as if you were the caregiver or parent of the hurt child (your inner child). No one understands her needs and sadness more than you. You are the best person to offer this apology to her. The following Apology Letter is an example.

STEP 5: ACKNOWLEDGE THE HURT

APOLOGY LETTER

Dear Marisa,

I am so sorry your father beat you with his army belt that bruised your tiny body. I am sorry you felt fearful at night and unsafe in your bed. I'm so sorry your father called you demeaning names, such as black sheep, stupid whore, and idiot, and that he told you that you would never amount to anything. I'm so sorry he disrespected you and didn't see how much pain he inflicted by his words and beatings. I am sorry he sexually abused you and that it caused you to fear and avoid intimacy. I am sorry it caused you to struggle in your relationships to the point you felt you were crazy. I am sorry your father was hateful and angry and directed his emotions onto you and caused you to hate him.

I am sorry your mother did not protect you or stop your father from hurting you. I am sorry your mother was fearful of your father and failed to keep you safe. I am sorry your brother was taught to disrespect you and find more ways for you to be punished. I'm sorry your father showed favouritism towards your sister and caused you to feel inadequate. I am sorry for the times your father pulled your hair and ears and hit you across the face while he yelled and belittled you. I'm sorry the pain and suffering continued for so many years without relief.

Please forgive me for what was done to you.

STEP 6: REMOVE THE GUILT AND BLAME

(Apology Letter continued)

Marisa, you did not deserve this inexcusable treatment. You are not guilty or to blame. This was not your fault. You are not bad, evil, or wrong as you thought you were.

STEP 7: Restitution—What Should Have Occurred

(Apology Letter continued)

Marisa, you deserved to be protected and loved. You deserved to be told you were beautiful and intelligent. You deserved to be hugged and kissed so that you felt valued. You deserved to know you were worthy of success and abundance. Your life should have been filled with compassion and kindness. You should have felt protected and supported, knowing you were precious. Your home and bed should have been a haven where you could rest, feel safe, grow and flourish. You should have known that you were perfect in every way.

STEP 8: Healing Thoughts and Imagery

Imagine the freedom of throwing your burdens away. Imagine the pain and suffering lifting from your body. Know that you can now surrender, trust, and free yourself. Imagine white and gold streaming light cleansing and dissolving your anger and resentment towards the person who hurt you. Decide to let go and allow the negativity to dissolve in the light. Choose to forgive. Let the angels heal your heart and heal the wounds so you can feel whole. See the past behind you and choose to turn it in a new direction in order to become free in your life.

RESOURCE:

Click or copy the following link to play this special song called 'You're Free' http://marisarusso.com/youre-free/

STEP 9: FORGIVE YOURSELF

Just as you completed the Apology process for someone else, if you harbour guilt and shame for your own past, repeat steps 5-8 to forgive yourself.

STEP 10: REVIEW YOUR ANGER RATING

Rate your current feeling of hurt now towards the person you identified in the previous steps. On a scale of one to ten — ten being the most intense anger, zero being none. Your anger level may feel reduced, replaced with feelings of relief and peace.

When I reflect on what others have endured it often causes me sadness. These are times I feel a strong need to apologise for many injustices that have been done to them. One of them is to black and indigenous people, so I wrote this poem to express my feelings and to apologise for their cruel history.

SORRY POEM TO BLACK PEOPLE

My dearest black friend,
I'm sorry for the inhumanity
It's not your fault, it was insanity
I am sorry for your suffering and pain
I am sorry for the years of shackles and chains
I seek forgiveness and I ask for your mercy
It's the same as Joan of Arc, who was tried for
    heresy
I know your suffering was relentless
There was no law to stop the madness

The Bible said that Cain killed Abel
And then, God created a curse, a fairy tale fable
He punished Cain by marking him black
This gave man permission to torture without facts
There's a great injustice to your children,
    mothers, and fathers
Your soul has been void of feeling love from others
Who gave man the right to own a human life and
    force slavery on your people?
Your hearts have bled from pain, suffering, and
    maltreatment
Is there a place that holds willingness?
That I may in humility receive your forgiveness?
The Earth and its children can have peace and
    true victory
Can you release me from the damage to your
    history?

I seek your permission to free this karmic debt
The Earth has been suffering and under threat
It was your spiritual powers that sealed your fate
It was this greatness that created the hate
If only you knew how brightly you shine
If only you knew how your worth is divine
Please forgive me for seeking this plight
I just want your forgiveness, your blessing and
    your light

PRACTICE THE APOLOGY AND HEALING STEPS 4-10

Practice steps 4 - 10 which can be completed on your own, or with another person. They allow you to give to yourself what you have been longing to receive in your life. The words fill a void and release the burdens and guilt to restore your self-worth, dignity, self-respect, and love. It is a powerful process that will shift your energy field. Feeling different — being different — will then shift what you attract and experience. When pain and suffering are removed from your energy field, you attract less pain and suffering. When anger is released, the same rule applies. These exercises can be repeated many times for different people and experiences in your life.

Take charge of nurturing and healing yourself. You have earned and deserve healing and so much more.

Chapter 5:
PATTERNS

THE AUCTION

I first met John in the Mormon temple about a year after I returned from Canada to Australia. I wasn't in a hurry to involve myself in another relationship, as I wasn't certain I could make one work, yet I felt an instant attraction to him. The relationship came with some unwanted baggage: a vindictive ex-wife and custody court battles. This did not help our relationship as I was already emotionally and physically struggling in my own life. Even though our initial attraction didn't last, we were two people who understood each other, and we made it work for the most part of our marriage.

John sat silently unperturbed, as I paced the wooden floors, listening to the auctioneer's pleas for someone to give an opening bid on our house. One month before, we had purchased our dream home in a beautiful seaside location and now we were trying to sell our current house to pay for it. As I peeked through the crack to the outside, I saw beads of sweat pouring down the auctioneer's face as he attempted to draw an offer from the unmoved group of people standing in front of him. We soon surmised that the twenty-strong crowd had no intention of placing any bids. The crowd consisted of nosey neighbours, curious onlookers, and tyre kickers. I wondered why the heck they would turn up to watch us fail miserably to get an offer for our beloved home. Didn't they have better things to do?

The moment I walked into our new house, I felt peaceful; the peacock that magically appeared on the back doorstep was our confirmation it was the house for us. John calculated our ability to pay the new mortgage by selling our current house at the market price of the previous four weeks, and factored in that we needed a 20% increase in our business sales.

Unfortunately, quickly after we signed the mortgage papers for our new house, interest rates rose twice in eight weeks. Simultaneously, the real estate market took a dramatic decline and house prices dropped rapidly. I was in a huge panic as the predicament we had just created meant there was a high probability we could lose everything.

Now house buyers were on the hunt, looking for bargains from vulnerable homeowners who were caught in similar situations to ours — under pressure to sell their home at any price they could get. Even our low opening bid was not low enough to attract an offer.

We thought we had done everything to keep the energy positive for a smooth transaction. We chose a friendly and reputable agent to represent us. We burned aromatic oils, cleared the house of negativity with my healing techniques, and on top of all of that, we visualised the house being sold, and created a vision board with the sold sticker on our house. We used every conceivable law of attraction and ritual method we knew to get the house sold. However, it did not seem to matter what we did, as luck was not on our side, or at least it seemed that way.

The auction was passed in with zero bids, and defeat was written all over the auctioneer's face as he entered the house, looking dishevelled. "They're a tough crowd," he said, wiping his brow.

This is not a good outcome, I thought. My mind raced as I starting scanning all possible solutions to pay the two mortgages we now had, on two houses that had devalued in price.

As I thought through options to solve our crisis, none of the solutions seemed like workable scenarios. All I could see was my own blood, sweat, and tears from decades of hard work all coming to an end. The worst part was that my "hard earned" dollars that had paid for our house felt like exactly that. Each dollar I earned consisted of physical suffering I had endured over decades of my working career. Many of those days, months, and years I had wished away, as I suffered in so much physical pain and exhaustion.

After the auctioneer and crowd left, I continued to pace the wooden floors, feeling extremely vulnerable. I wondered how it turned out so wrong since we followed our feelings, which I thought should lead to positive outcomes. Fearful of not being able to control any aspect of the real estate market, I started mentally playing the "what if" game. It made me realise how much I yearned for peace and freedom. I had the desire to escape to a sunny, deserted island with no possessions, feeling totally free in mind and spirit. Alas, it was only a dream and not my reality.

I was afraid that I would have to spend my life paying off a large financial debt, while still living with physical pain, depression, chronic fatigue, and not have anything to show for it. I felt imprisoned with no solution to the problem. The dilemma consumed my thoughts and my stress levels were high. I was at the point I didn't want to talk about other people's problems or watch anything negative on TV. My energy was so fragile; I knew that if I heard any more bad stories I would fall to pieces. I had a yearning to be around kind, positive people who told kind, positive stories.

Knowing I couldn't live with the stress of the situation for much longer, I was forced to surrender to the outcome. I had been trying to placate myself by saying if I got through the situation without losing everything, then I would never worry about anything again. Even though only material possessions were at risk, I couldn't see myself starting over again. I didn't have the energy, or the willpower, to rebuild my life. My insecurity triggered memories of all the previous times I had been without money. I had never wanted to feel so vulnerable again, yet here I was on the same merry-go-round.

I forced myself to repeat the affirmation "It always works out, it always does," and reminded myself I had survived my childhood and other helpless situations.

During many of those dark times, I felt as if angels stepped into my path to help me. I had a positive pattern and a belief that things do eventually work out, so I was counting on this positive pattern to come to fruition.

The upshot of this story is we survived without financial loss. Along the way, there were many twists and turns to beat the odds of what we were up against. We rented our unsaleable house and moved into our new beachside home. It was a rollercoaster ride to say the least, as we tried unsuccessfully a couple more times to sell while we struggled to pay both mortgages. Despite this, John and I were risk takers and we both agreed that we needed to invest money in our business and ourselves in order to make more money. We stretched ourselves to the maximum and invested a large amount in touring the USA, hoping the outcome would be a profitable return.

Overall, we were continually paying off a huge debt, our credit cards were at their limits, and our accounts were in overdraft. Despite our increase in business sales and our apparent success, we couldn't shake the feeling of heaviness. Our downfall was in employing people with hidden agendas. I missed the betrayal signs that they were subtly showing because I was under a lot of pressure.

The entire journey stretched me personally *and* professionally more than any other time in my life. I felt the strain to become a better healer as John tripled my healing session fees. Even though I protested, it forced me to become a better therapist. We challenged ourselves to produce great healing products and it was during those years I recorded a lot of the DVD courses available today. It was almost like we were put into a difficult financial situation to push us to create our greatest outcome, the Forensic Healing System, which has since won three Australian Achievers awards and is changing lives worldwide.

The entire experience has given me a profound understanding of the power of energy and why negative and positive situations occur in our lives. *Nothing can replace personal experience.* I have personally experienced and applied every principle I teach. I now recognise most of the stressful situations in my life as the "vulnerability" pattern that followed me for years.

In the Forensic Healing System, I teach how to identify patterns in your adult life that stem from childhood traumas and negative experiences. My pattern stemmed from childhood, as I consistently felt vulnerable to outside influences such as my father's abuse. I felt I had no control over his actions, which left me feeling trapped in a place I could not leave. This created a fear of being vulnerable and ultimately drew similar scenarios to me, as what you fear, you create. It has taken my whole life to overcome this pattern that was my norm, my basic belief about life.

My father's betrayal left me vulnerable to his abusive behaviour. This created a consistent pattern of attracting other deceitful people who would betray me. Now, I can acknowledge my patterns and what I needed to do to change. I can trust, surrender and believe that everything will work out. I no longer operate in the same manner. I no longer make unconscious decisions that set me up for being trapped and vulnerable. I now make very deliberate and careful decisions.

You will have your own familiar patterns with others as you do the same dance each time you interact with them. I see the same common negative patterns with women and their partners. The most familiar pattern is the women feel their partners are negative, blaming, and disrespectful towards them. They feel hurt, undervalued, and victimised, yet nothing seems to change in their relationships. The process of changing patterns is to become aware that you are the common denominator in the relationships. Even though you may leave a bad relationship, you may find you end up in a similar relationship, with similar problems. The problem is taking the same "you" with you.

READING THE PATTERNS

Everything reveals itself in patterns. Relationships, finances, and health and spiritual conditions all exhibit patterns – both good and bad. Identifying and eliminating the predominant negative patterns that hold you back, allows new patterns to be created. These negative patterns are usually the most difficult to overcome and may seem impossible to change. If you really want a happier life, the universe designs negative life patterns so you will eventually realise that they cause you too much pain to hang on to them. The negative feelings act as a compass or guide so you can know *where* to redirect or change your life so it will become much more fulfilling.

REMEMBER: LIFE IS YOUR MESSAGE

These continual negative life patterns cause the stresses that have the most impact on your health. There are cases of clients who do everything to be healthy yet have so much emotional stress in their bodies, they barely function. There are also those who don't pay attention to being healthy, yet they have decided to live a carefree life and their health is still very good. Understanding your negative life patterns allows you to change your life to one of freedom and peacefulness.

EVERYTHING CONSISTS OF PATTERNS

Gregg Braden's book *The Divine Matrix* states that, "When something is holographic, it exists wholly within every fragment of itself, no matter how many pieces it's divided into." This illustration helps convey the idea that no matter how finely we divide the universe, each segment mirrors the whole universe, only on a smaller scale.

The same principle is conveyed in Michael Talbot's book *The Holographic Universe*, which provides supporting evidence of how our existence and experience can be viewed through a holographic model. This idea of the "whole" contained in each piece is the basis of the Holographic Principle.

David Wilcock's book *The Source Field Investigations* references the DNA "phantom effect experiment." This experiment entailed a strand of DNA being placed in a container with some random photons. The photons then created a structure around the DNA. The DNA was then removed from the container, and the photons stayed in the same pattern as the DNA. Further experiments confirmed that when the container was removed, the photons stayed in exactly the same place without the container. The pattern of photons remained in place for approximately thirty days.

We can therefore conclude that our DNA leaves an imprint and attracts particles to it that can become a physical form. Since everyone leaves a trail of themselves everywhere they go, having a good trail of DNA is important for our energy field.

PATTERNS IN OUR CONNECTIONS WITH OTHERS

What does it mean when people say, "We are all connected"? There are no physical ties to other people, or are there? Science has some interesting experiments to demonstrate that we are connected through the source field.

Just as the photons mimicked the single strand of DNA, human beings do the same. For instance, when we sit in a chair, we leave an energetic imprint of ourselves from our DNA. This energy can have an influence on the next person who sits in the chair. We are continually walking through energetic imprints and leaving our own DNA energetic imprints. This is most apparent when you walk into a room with very loving and happy people. The vibrations and imprints uplift you and change how you feel. It can create feelings of happiness and peacefulness even though words may not be exchanged.

This may explain how the art of psychometry works. Psychometry is a psychic or intuitive ability in which a person can sense or "read" the history of an object by touching it. The reading entails disclosing details of the person who owned the object without ever meeting or knowing them. The reader receives impressions in forms of images, sounds, smells, tastes, and emotions.

When you think about the significance of this research — it confirms that we have the potential to influence our surroundings — it shows that we must, positively and constructively, become one with each other. We must recognise that our energy, emotions, and actions are influencing and affecting others and the planet, more than we realise. We are shaping and creating the world we live in. The "shift" is now occurring for everyone to become unified and supportive of each other. *Competing* with others is no longer effective for the new energies that are emerging. Old, corrupt systems that neglect the planet, animals, and people are collapsing and being replaced by new systems that restore humanity and unite people.

Even though the world seems to have a frightening and unstable future, this instability has caused many spiritual changes in people. It has challenged and pushed people to look *within* themselves to find peace and strength to contend with the outside world and the changes happening to the planet. This prompts an evolution of creating a much more peaceful and brighter world. This is the emerging world and we can create it with our intentions, actions, and vibrations. Each and every one of us is a co-creator of our lives and the world in which we live.

FREEING WOMEN EXERCISE:
CHANGING YOUR PATTERNS

- Find the cause of your patterns and identify them.
- Find the message your patterns are teaching you.
- Focus on achieving what you want.
- Create a plan to react differently in your relationships.

STEP 11: FINDING YOUR NEGATIVE LIFE PATTERN

A) Make a list of the three most stressful situations you've experienced in your life (not including your childhood). They are most likely based on relationship problems. Write down your feelings in each situation.

B) Analyse the "Hurt Letter" written from Step 1 in Chapter 3. Identify the common theme that has been repeated in your adult life from childhood. Find the similarities of circumstances and feelings that are repeated and write down your findings.

Choose one predominant pattern below that matches the information you have found in the previous two exercises; A and B. Write down only one of the following 18 patterns — the one that is most consistent to your findings. When you change your predominant pattern, you start changing the other patterns.

1. **Distrust:** You have struggled to trust others as you have felt so betrayed that trusting is very challenging to do. *Opposite: to feel trust.*

2. **Grief:** You have experienced a lot of grief and this feeling has constantly weighed you down with a heavy heart. *Opposite: to feel whole and healed.*

3. **Guilt:** You have felt guilty about situations. You agree to do things only because you feel obligated and you think it is the "right" thing to do. *Opposite: to feel free and innocent.*

4. **Hopelessness:** You have been in very grim circumstances. You have felt you have been in a black hole of despair with no way out. *Opposite: to feel hope and optimism.*

5. **Hurt:** You have experienced deep hurt from other people who have betrayed you. This feels ingrained on your heart and has manifested as a feeling of heaviness and emotional pain. *Opposite: to feel healed and respected.*

6. **Insecurity:** Your life has felt insecure. You seek to control it so you can feel safe and secure. You avoid taking risks or making big changes in your life. *Opposite: to feel safe, whole, and secure.*

7. **Judgement:** Your self-talk has been very negative and others judge you. You have judged yourself and others harshly. *Opposite: to feel accepted and loved unconditionally.*

8. **Letting Go:** You have hung on to negative experiences or people. You have thought about them so often it affects your life. *Opposite: to feel unburdened and release bad memories.*

9. **Purposelessness:** You have searched and struggled to know what your life purpose is without ever finding it. *Opposite: to feel purpose and passion.*

10. **Overwhelmed:** Your life experiences have felt so overwhelming that you have wanted to give up on life. *Opposite: to feel peace and calm.*

11. **Potential:** Circumstances have made it difficult for you to reach your full potential. It has been a continuous struggle for you to live your passions. *Opposite: to feel progression and uniqueness.*

12. **Powerlessness:** You have given your power away and others upset you easily. You have made decisions based on what others think. You have felt you have had no control of your life. *Opposite: to feel empowered and confident.*

13. **Relationships:** You have struggled in your relationships and your close relationships seem difficult. This stretches your relationship skills, and improves them so you respond in a calm and assertive manner. *Opposite: to feel harmony and support in your relationships.*

14. **Sacrifice:** You have put yourself last in everything. Your self-worth has come from serving others. You have felt worn out due to the daily grind of giving and never receiving. *Opposite: to feel nurtured and valued.*

15. **Trapped:** You have felt stuck in your life. Others have trapped you into circumstances you do not want. *Opposite: to feel free and energised.*

16. **Vulnerability:** You have been hurt in the past and you fear being hurt again. You have put up emotional barriers that disconnect you from people. *Opposite: to feel safe and connected.*

17. **Victimised:** Unfair things have been done to you or you have been a victim of other people or situations. You have felt you had no choices in life. *Opposite: to feel empowered and respected.*

18. Worthlessness: You have never felt validated as a person. People have put you down and made you feel inferior or not good enough. *Opposite: to feel worthy and loved.*

FINDING THE MESSAGE YOUR PATTERNS ARE TEACHING YOU

The predominant pattern you identified will have an opposite, positive pattern on which you need to focus. The opposite pattern is written with the Negative Life Pattern. For example, my Negative Life Pattern was being vulnerable. The opposite pattern for me to focus on and create was to feel safe and connected. When I analyse my adult life, I can see how I set myself up to be in many vulnerable situations by not thinking things through and analysing all the risks. I was not aware I was repeating my patterns — therefore I continually made mistakes.

Write answers to Steps 12 - 14 in your journal. In the following examples my negative life pattern was vulnerability and the opposite, positive pattern is feeling safe and connected.

STEP 12: THE MESSAGE FROM YOUR PATTERNS

What Message have you learned from your negative pattern?

Example: **My message** is to make conscious decisions that are less risky, and to discontinue relationships with people who show signs of betrayal.

STEP 13: YOUR NEW FOCUS

What will be your Focus? What do you want to feel and create?

Example: **My focus** is to feel safe and secure, and create relationships with trustworthy and honest people.

STEP 14: YOUR PLAN

What is your Plan to create a positive pattern?

Example: **My plan** is to analyse the signs that people who are not trustworthy show, be clearer about what I want in a relationship, be more thorough analysing my risks, and connecting so I can feel if things are right for me.

CHAPTER 6:
SELFISH

I felt as though I had been living my whole life in a coma and just woke up. It was two weeks after I received an unexpected healing for a sacrifice vow removal. This entailed a deep energy healing where I struggled to breathe as I affirmed the words to release a vow or contract that kept me in hardship and suffering.

I had been studying kinesiology and met with another skilled energy healer who identified the vow and channelled energy for the vow to be released. For any onlooker, it would appear the healing entailed words, statements, and touching points on the body. However for me, it was very tangible as my body reacted with pulsating energy running through it, physically causing my body to arch and struggle for air as I attempted to release the programming that was etched deep into my cells.

When the sacrifice vow was finally removed, I burst into tears from relief. The release left me feeling like a two-ton truck had hit me. I felt tired, dazed, and disconnected. It took two weeks to finally recover and feel connected again. In the moment of full recovery I stood in the middle of the lounge room wondering; *what the hell was I thinking?*

This was the moment I realised with true clarity that I had been setting myself up to play the martyr. You know, the one who says, "Let me take the hit, someone has to do it." In fact, I must have been well on my way to being canonised as a saint when I realised I had fought and cared for every underdog that came my way. I was committed to taking on other's hardships, along with my own. I think I should have been locked up for my own personal safety. Now, I am happy to say, martyrdom is definitely on its way out, no longer the trend it was in Biblical times. However it is still a pattern all too common with the women I encounter.

I recalled flashes of the times I tried to help people in need and was rewarded with big fat kick up the backside in the form of hurt and betrayal. *Holy cow!* I thought. Every choice I had made lead to hardship and suffering. This idea had never occurred to me two weeks prior, or at any other time in my life. Even though I said I wanted an easy and happy life, I was spiritually and emotionally compelled to make decisions that seemed I was "doing the right thing" or being a good person by focusing on others. Most of these decisions led to a mountain of suffering, sacrifice, and victimisation. If I divulged what some of them were, it would make you feel a whole lot better about your own life and decisions. Before I admit to any more "sins of stupidity," you need to recall in Chapter 3, I already pleaded guilty on the grounds of temporary insanity, so go easy on me!

When I was 26, I joined the Mormon Church in the amazing, romantic Italian city of Florence. I met a gorgeous Italian ophthalmologist called Marco. He was handsome, sexy, intelligent, funny, and he rocked my world. I believed I had met my true soul mate and every minute spent with him felt like magic. I felt safe, protected, loved, and passionate. We were inseparable and each knew what the other was thinking. He was the most encouraging man I had ever met and never spoke a critical word to me or to others. He believed I could do anything and his belief in me made me stronger than I thought was possible.

He joined the Mormon Church soon after I did. We spent a lot of time together, and we developed a romantic relationship. Marco eventually asked me to marry him and of course I responded with a big, fat, resounding YES. The Mormon Church teachings emphasised the importance of marrying in the church, so how perfect for me that Marco was now a Mormon. This meant that when Marco and I died, we could reach exaltation in the Celestial Kingdom or, in other words, hang out with JC, God himself, and other exalted beings. We would be living at the penthouse level in heaven.

Marco and I set a wedding date, and my mother and sister planned a trip to Florence from Australia to attend. I was very excited that I would finally engage in hot, passionate sex with a man I was madly in love with. As a fully-fledged Mormon, I was committed to the law of chastity so there was no hanky panky. Plus — I forgot to mention — I also gave up alcohol, drugs, cigarettes, tea, coffee, and swearing.

Spoiler alert: Marco decided to leave the Mormon Church a week before the wedding. I had an agonising choice to make. Should I marry him or should I stay faithful to what I thought at the time was the only true religion on Earth? My heart was torn and in my spiritual wisdom I chose not to marry Marco. Instead, I gathered the little money I had left and spent it serving a five-month Mormon mission in Rome with a broken heart. I then returned to Australia with no money, no husband, no future, and no passion — but at least I could say I was "dutiful and faithful" to my beliefs.

Then to top it all off, a bright idea was planted in my brain at the time I was still operating in "stupidity" mode. As I mingled with the Mormons, I listened to a story told by one of the leaders I admired. He described how he prayed to know Christ's suffering. Not long after he prayed, he was answered and fell into a deep depression with suicidal tendencies that lasted three years. When I heard the story, I thought, *what a good idea, I am going to pray for the same thing!* And so I did. After all, I had nothing else to do since I was no longer getting married.

Are you yelling yet? I hear you, okay, and I could shock you even more. When I finally did get married to my first (Canadian) husband, it was beyond bad. So bad I don't want to lead you into a three-year depression by giving you the gory details. I think you get the picture and maybe you can relate to me when you ponder your own past decisions.

I have come out of my "stupidity" and "temporary insanity" states. I am now a fully-fledged empowered woman who settles for nothing less than an abundance of people and situations that support and nurture her. My tolerance to anything less is zero, and life has never worked better for me.

Life delivers exactly what you think you are worth and your worth is reflected in the choices you make.

THE REASONS: CONDITIONING

I am going to talk about something you may not realise is affecting many aspects of your life: the dreaded "R" word — Religion — which will give you some food for thought to move forward.

There is an undercurrent of energy that has been working against you — and all women — for centuries. I am well versed in the Biblical scriptures; I was born a Catholic and became a faithful member of the Mormon Church for eighteen years. I spent most of those years studying and teaching the scriptures, keeping myself "worthy." *Now* I recognise I had no self-worth and was trying to prove my worth by my faithfulness and Godliness. My missionary experience included meeting other members from other religions and I realised they all have one thing in common. No religion is in agreement or congruent with their interpretation of the scriptures. They all have their own spin on what "God" was trying to tell us.

I have no spin on any of the meanings in the scriptures. I take them at face value. There is no hidden meaning and there is no mistaking what the Bible teaches. I will show you how the words in the Bible have dictated your worth, respect, and recognition on a global level. For some poor women this has had devastating and deadly effects. Knowledge is power and education gives you tools to be successful. Women have been denied this opportunity and now I am going to explain the facts behind all of the subtle conditioning that has set the scene for global consciousness of your worth.

LIFE IS A SCIENCE

The Bible has consistently ranked as the world's number one bestseller and is the most widely distributed book in the world — an estimated *five billion* copies have been printed during the past 200 years.

Approximately a third of the world's population is Christian. Judaism and Islam also regard the Old Testament as part of their sacred scriptures. So, in essence, every day, one in three people makes choices that align with religious beliefs, attend religious groups or indoctrinate themselves and their children into the teachings in whichever rendition of the holy books they deem most authoritative.

The enormity of these teachings is the anchor to many prejudices — one of them being prejudice towards women. As I explain the significance of Biblical scriptures (which represent the word of God, the ultimate lawmaker) you will see how the words in the Bible have become a reality. These writings have set you up for disempowerment from the day you were born.

This religious conditioning has become an invisible, powerful force that has created a global consciousness and belief system. It influences every person at some level. You don't have to be religious or read the scriptures to be affected; it seeps into the psyche of every man, woman, and child.

It pains me to read what the Bible and other religious texts say about women. Labelling women (alternately) as evil and guilty. The Bible and Qur'an condone the abuse of women, which explains where women derive their low self-worth and sense of guilt. How have Bible references become a living reality in your own life or the lives of others? Here are just a few examples:

GENESIS 3:16: Eve (woman) is cursed with painful childbirth and domination by husband.

"Unto the woman he said, I will greatly multiply thy sorrow and thy conception. In sorrow thou shalt bring forth children: and thy desire shall be to thy husband, and he shall rule over thee."

EXODUS 21: 4: Wife and children are master's (husband's) property.

"If his master has given him a wife, and she has borne him sons or daughters, the wife and her children shall be her master's, and he shall go out by himself."

EXODUS 22:18: Commandment to kill witches (or women deemed evil).

"Thou shalt not suffer a witch to live."

1 TIMOTHY 2:11: Women are to be silent and submissive.

"Let the woman learn in silence with all subjection."

These scriptures are considered to be the word of God! These are just a few of the sobering scriptures that demonstrate the promotion of abuse and discrimination toward women. There is more detail in the Bible on how to kill, torture, and abuse women and children. If these scriptures exist in the *number one bestselling book*, and the law of attraction states, "words become thoughts and thoughts become things," what have patriarchal scribes created via the scriptures?

You may be thinking that you are not religious and this does not affect you. However, the trans-generational repetitions of these teachings, embedded in DNA have created an undercurrent of belief. I've estimated that over 30% of the world's population (approximately 2.5 billion people) vibrate to these messages, both consciously and unconsciously.

The Bible states that the creation of something begins with the word (John 1:1 "In the beginning was the Word, and the Word was with God, and the Word was God.") Let me explain this concept more clearly.

RESOURCE:

Read my full manifesto at http://marisarusso.com
Download the Women Breaking Free eBook

THE POWER OF THOUGHT

Lynne McTaggart is an author and researcher who investigates ways to change social behaviours and consciousness. The subjects in her experiments focus simultaneously on one issue at a given time, for a given duration.

In 2008, Lynne conducted a "Peace Intention Experiment" consisting of 12,000 participants who focused peaceful thoughts on Sri Lanka. The result? Lynne found a 74% reduction in violence after the experiment. Currently, there are more than 25 scientifically controlled, web-based experiments to test the power of thought to change the physical world. They have measured how group thought affects the growth of plants, polluted water, and lowering of violence in war-torn areas.

TIME TO WAKE UP

These experiments demonstrate that people with focused intentions can create or change conditions. If we can motivate people to "intend" peace, humanity, and healing, we can create a more humane world. There is a continuing effort to change the world by shifting consciousness or world thinking. However, I believe the Bible and other scripture are like the sandbags that hold down an air balloon to keep it from taking flight. People need to start thinking for themselves and incorporate decisions based on humanity and integrity. It begins with you and me, one leader and one neighbourhood at a time.

HISTORY HAS IT'S SCARS

Over the course of three centuries in modern Europe and in 17th-century America, women with healing gifts were burned, drowned, hung, tortured, and condemned as evil during "witch-hunts." There were many reasons for being accused of being a witch, including being clever, having a face-mole, being intuitive, or being clairvoyant. Other reasons included the use of herbs, an inability to bear children, or a husband who chose to have an affair or died before his wife did!

What was the purpose? I believe the purpose of suppressing women was to shut down their innate spiritual powers and intuition. I believe the subjugation of women is deeply embedded in worldwide beliefs and global consciousness.

WHO HAS THE ANSWERS?

- The majority of world leaders and politicians are men.
- The majority of worldwide companies have male CEOs and senior management.
- The majority of women earn lower wages on average than men with similar qualifications.
- Why did laws exist to prohibit women from working and exclude them from education?
- Why do some countries prohibit women from voting?

- Why are the vast majority of abusers male?
- Why did UK family law give husbands ownership of their wives and children (a wife was deemed property), make it lawful to beat them, and inherit all their finances and assets?
- Why did the churches facilitate kidnappings of unwed women's babies?
- Why did the churches torture, burn, and drown innocent women and children whom they called witches?
- Why are the majority of controlling and abusive cults and religions run by men?
- Why do some women marry their rapist to reduce humiliation and shame?
- Why does China and India support female infanticide and sex selection for boys?

Some extreme cases still exist in the Middle East and Africa:

- Why do Egyptian courts require women to lose all their financial assets and prove abuse if they want a divorce?
- Why do some Middle East laws not criminalise rape and allow husbands ownership of their wives' bodies?
- Why do men in Saudi Arabia brutally maim women if they don't wear a burqa (covering her face and body)?
- Why does the Moroccan penal code of women's rape determine the penalty by rating the victim's sexual experience?
- Why does the horror of female genital mutilation still exist today?
- Why do some husbands torture and kill their wives and call it an honour killing?
- Why do some African cultures encourage men and their families to beat their wives?

These are disturbing situations and questions with no legitimate answers. This unacceptable behaviour needs to stop. The goal of this book is to shift your energy field by changing your beliefs and thoughts about *your worth and sacredness*. These conditions for women can change when the global consciousness changes. I am passionate about assisting with these changes and helping to create new possibilities for you and for women in general.

WHO'S YOUR IDOL?

I was 26 when I was baptised into the Mormon Church, signifying that I agreed to follow the teachings of Jesus. I was fully submerged in water to cleanse my sins and oblige myself to follow Christ in the Mormon faith. This, in essence, contracted me to a life of suffering, service, poverty, hardship, and obedience. A lifelong servitude to the Church and its God. I was told that my reward would be in heaven. So I became a proud, suffering Mormon.

I was constantly told, "Where much is given, much is required." In other words, my lot in life was to pay for my sins through suffering and to pay my debt to Christ for sacrificing his life for me. I wondered why, over the centuries, the debt to Christ had not been paid off? I now believe that Mormonism is somewhat similar to Scientology and the billion-year contract their members (including children) sign to commit their soul to an eternity of service to the faith. I believe these types of contracts and vows keep souls bound, lifetime after lifetime — it makes sense that some people feel stuck in life.

One saintly role model is Mother Teresa, who has been quoted saying "I pray that I may always know suffering so that I may know God." Christopher Hitchens' book on her life, *The Missionary Position*, claims she would often deny medication to the sick, as she believed that suffering was their spiritual journey back to God.

My mother was an influential role model. By putting herself last, she conditioned me to also place my needs last, and ignore my feelings. When I was baptised twice, I made contracts to follow Jesus. One with the Catholic Church and one with the Mormon Church. The ritual of baptism bound me to Christian living. When I experienced the healing to remove the sacrifice vows, it removed some deeply etched contracts in my soul that kept me living a life of martyrdom and sacrifice.

WHAT IS SACRIFICE?

There are many types of sacrifice that have made history and we make sacrifices on a daily basis in our lives. I believe that sacrifice means there is a cost involved to do something. For instance, if a person voluntarily pays for another person's expenses, even though the person paying doesn't have the money to give, then it is a sacrifice. If a wealthy person paid the expenses, there is less of a sacrifice as his or her financial status is not affected, and it doesn't create hardship.

I've witnessed women who too often sacrifice themselves by tolerating negative and disrespectful behaviour. They've been conditioned to believe that they should send love and blessings even to those who are hateful or abusive to them. Emotion is energy, so I say, "Give your love and blessings to those who earn it. Don't give the gift of love to someone who abuses or disrespects you; there are many deserving people who will appreciate your kindness. Give your love to those who want it so you feel appreciated rather than taken for granted and disrespected."

Women often base their self-worth on their ability to help others. This belief runs very strongly in people who have low self-worth. Mothers do this consistently. They put their children's needs first, and never have time for themselves. This continues the cycle of teaching their daughters to do the same.

ARE YOU ASKING FOR THE WRONG THINGS?

We all sacrifice ourselves to some degree; we all exhibit some tendency to give of ourselves to our own detriment. Ponder these questions:

- Do you feel used after you have given?
- Do you give to others before you give to yourself?
- Do you fight other people's battles?

If you answered yes to any of these questions, that would indicate you compromise yourself. We learn in religious teachings to be like Christ. You need to suffer or you need to give and serve to feel worthy. This may then lead to feelings of guilt if you spend time on your own comfort or enjoyment.

If you don't love, respect, and value yourself, then the universe can't deliver your desires. If you feel unworthy of receiving, or you think your value comes from giving to others, this is sending a message of unworthiness. Simple signs may include when you get held up on the phone listening to a complaining friend who never asks about your needs. Or when you constantly agree to your partner's needs, and rarely make your own needs known. The universe is always responding to your *vibration*. It matches this vibration and gives you more ways to serve and to try to fill the void of not being enough.

SUFFERING BOB

Bob considered himself to be a spiritual man. When his wife was dying in hospital from bowel cancer he was angry with the doctors. He felt they were negligent and inflicted more harm than good. He looked worn out and weary. His wife eventually died, which led him to book a consultation to see me. He said he tried to heal himself but was getting nowhere and he was at his wits' end.

When he lay on the treatment table, I asked him to explain his relationship with Jesus. He said that he believed in his mission. I asked him to give more detail of what that meant. He replied it meant following Jesus' ways: being kind to one another and serving our fellow man. I commented that he was a great Christ follower. Bob was living the same life as JC, as it consisted of suffering, poverty, sacrifice, service, and heading for an unhappy ending. *This was Bob's epiphany.* He looked at me in bewilderment, and then replied that it was true, he was just like Christ but without the fame or a book!

WHAT MESSAGES ARE YOU LAUNCHING INTO THE UNIVERSE?

When you make the choice of putting yourself last, you send out a message that you don't care about yourself. Each time you make a choice to please someone else or give at your expense, you tell the universe that your needs don't matter, so the universe says, "OK, I will give you even more experiences that show you that you don't matter."

This causes more resentment and attracts more negative experiences. This can keep you stuck in a cycle. I can hear you argue that I am asking you to be selfish. The word "selfish" has negative connotations and is associated with bad people who are uncaring and think only of themselves. This causes you to lean in the other direction so you are never accused of being selfish, as that would affect your already low self-worth. Just think of selfish as *self-care,* and get over the fact that your job is no longer to look after everyone else. Your new job description is putting yourself first as you will begin to realise that nobody else is putting you first. The following true story about my school friend, will explain.

MELISSA'S MUM

Melissa didn't always have it easy growing up, losing her father and brother and being raised by her single mother. However, she seemed to deal with whatever was thrown at her. She was the wise one who would tell you what to do in any given circumstance. She enjoyed life, and in our early twenties we met up in foreign countries to travel and have fun adventures together.

Recently I visited her in her home in an affluent Melbourne suburb in Australia. She looked fit, trim, and terrific. It seemed things hadn't changed much as she was still jet-setting around the world, living a life that most could only dream of. Melissa walked me through her newly renovated house. Her handsome husband was at work earning a healthy living and her lovely boys resembled Prince Harry and Prince William.

As we began to chat, I asked her to describe her mother. She responded that she would have been considered "selfish" as she did things to please herself. This response gave me the insight to her amazing life. Just as her mother chose to do things to make herself happy, Melissa instinctively made choices in her life that were beneficial and supportive of a great lifestyle. She made career choices that would support her love of travel, she chose a man to marry who ticked all the boxes, she maintained friendships with fun, outgoing people who respected her. She kept herself healthy and fit by going to the gym regularly. She rarely made any decisions that were detrimental or sacrificial. End result: a very balanced, wonderful life!

What has your mother taught you?

FREEING WOMEN EXERCISE:
CANCEL CONTRACTS, VOWS AND OBLIGATIONS

STEP 15: YOUR MOTHER/CARER'S SACRIFICIAL BEHAVIOUR

Make a list of the ways your mother/carer has sacrificed or devalued herself.

STEP 16: YOUR SACRIFICIAL BEHAVIOUR

Make a list of ways you sacrifice or devalue yourself.

STEP 17: YOUR SACRIFICIAL SIGNS

Make a list of symbols or reminders of your sacrifice.

For example: Search around your house and gather the items that signify sacrifice, service, stress, or suffering. This will include such things as:

- Religious pictures
- Baptismal certificate
- Rosary beads
- Pictures of ex-lovers that broke your heart or hurt you
- Furniture or clothes that are associated with bad memories

- Gifts from people who betrayed you
- Childhood memorabilia, if your childhood was difficult
- Letters or documents that remind you of problems and stress

I highly recommend that you remove these items or put them in a box and store them in the garage so they are out of sight and away from your energy field. You will be surprised how much better you will feel. Enjoy the sensation of the weight of these obligations and past troubles being lifted off your shoulders.

STEP 18: FREEING WOMEN'S ACTIVATION

If you are itching to get rid of any conditioning that has bound you in the past, you're in luck, as I have created a free healing activation that reverses the control and conditioning of women. It releases the subtle manipulations, detrimental contracts and doctrines from religious texts, guilty feelings, and sacrificial patterns that have bound you in persecution, poverty, suffering, and low self-worth.

It includes a powerful energetic healing as I direct healing energies for you to reclaim your birthright, freedom, and divinity, so you can experience more than you ever thought possible. It returns your sacredness, value, equality, and spiritual powers that in turn will heal our children and Mother Earth. It is a step into freedom and my most significant creation to date. To formalise the process, after your activation you will receive a personalised certificate to symbolise your new declaration of freedom.

RESOURCE:

The Freeing Women Activation is free at http://marisarusso.com/fug-reader/

WAKING UP

When you recognise that feeling happy, free, and fulfilled will change everything in your life for the better, you will no longer compromise yourself. Whether my current situation of being highly sensitive and susceptible to others' energy is fortunate or unfortunate, it has caused me to make changes in my life so that I am diligent and constantly keep the energy around me in check. I resemble a person who has chronic food allergies and knows the consequences of eating the wrong foods. It is no different to me with energy. I have trained myself to be a clear, open conduit to channel energy to heal others; therefore, I am also open to emotions, thoughts and intentions, and agendas of others. Just as people have strict diets, I have strict emotional boundaries with others out of necessity.

CHAPTER 7:
POWER

All the mistakes ever made in the world have been repeatedly made by millions of people. I've noticed more people seem to fail rather than succeed in life. With easy access to helpful information, *everyone* should be a success story. Surely someone has cracked the real success formula by now? It seems there are more books written on how to succeed in life than there are people on fad diets!

So what's going on? Where's the *real* manual that explains the secrets of life and how to avoid making repetitive mistakes? This chapter gives you the formula that drives people's success, as most people are unaware of the energy exchanges that fuel their outcomes. These concepts will alter your own disempowering behaviour, and cause you to scrutinise yourself and the people with whom you surround yourself.

The odds were stacked against me to succeed in life. My foundation was an abusive upbringing with limited family support and then some of my peers and colleagues spent years trying to push me down. Despite the setbacks, I am now highly successful and can attribute my ongoing success to the concepts I openly share. You are going to discover how to access as much power as you need to succeed in any area of your life.

THE SINKING OF THE TITANIC

This knowledge became apparent when I made one particular mistake, which was humiliating to say the least. It felt like my worst nightmare of being butt naked in front of a crowd, ready to die of embarrassment. The only difference was not waking up in relief, thinking I didn't have to leave town or find new friends.

The nightmare occurred on a cold Sunday afternoon in my home city many years ago, where I was preparing to give a healing demonstration to 250 people. I was familiar with the format and procedures for the day. All my prior demonstrations had been successful enough for me to continue doing them, and they consistently attracted new students to become Forensic Healers. This time was very different and was a powerful teaching moment that could have severely affected my healing and therapy career.

I was presenting in a large conference room to some loyal followers. The remainder of the audience was a large group of people I had never met, having responded to an advertisement inviting them to a free healing demonstration. As we began to set up for the demonstration, one thing after another went wrong.

First we discovered we were missing cords for our computer, and the cord I hurriedly purchased didn't fit. The venue didn't inform us they were renovating making it difficult to access and there was wet sand along the pathway that people walked through to enter. People arrived late and left early. The staff assisting that day were distracting as they chatted with each other during my presentation. Some of the audience members sat facing me with folded arms with the words "prove yourself" were flashing like a neon sign across their forehead. Not a very inviting group to present to!

I got the message loud and clear. The positive flow that I was accustomed to was definitely out the window.

When I begin any demonstration, I ask the audience as to whether they believe in the law of attraction. I explain that it is essentially the concept that emotions or feelings you give out come back to you, and draw people in similar situations to yourself. On that day, barely anyone from the audience raised a hand. It took me by surprise that the group I was about to present to did not believe in the law of attraction, and it seemed their intent was to prove me wrong.

I was accustomed to seeing the majority of a group raise their hands and very few (if any) would not be familiar with the law of attraction concept taught by the amazing Esther Hicks. I had no idea it would affect the result of my presentation. I just thought that it would be an interesting experience — *"interesting"* now being an understatement.

Everything went downhill from that point. No one who volunteered to receive a healing was experiencing any change in pain levels. Although I can address any condition, I ask for volunteers experiencing pain, as the results are immediately noticeable.

My stress levels increased as I worked desperately on a female volunteer to direct healing energy to her arm and back. I could feel the energy coming through me the same way I felt in other healings. I could also see some of the audience reacting to the energy as they felt tingling sensations and some became teary and emotional. However, all eyes were still on the volunteer and me. After a couple of minutes the volunteer reported no changes in her pain levels. It was embarrassing and I did not know what to do. I tried to think smart, so I resorted to choosing a child to be the next volunteer. Children and animals are usually the easiest candidates for healings. Or so I thought!

I selected a fifteen-year-old boy and things just spiralled further downhill. Again I tried with as much energy as I could muster, but nothing changed the boy's head pain, which resulted from an operation many years prior. His father added that he was also a healer and nothing he or the medical profession did could relieve his son's pain.

Great, I thought, another person putting their limiting beliefs on me.

As the father was talking, I scanned the room for the nearest exit sign, which unfortunately was at the back of the room. I realised I was trapped at the front with all glaring eyes on me. I had never felt more disempowered and energetically sabotaged as I did in that moment. I looked down to the floor, secretly hoping to locate a hidden trap door through which I could disappear.

Following the boy, I asked for another volunteer to read their negative life pattern — the patterns previously mentioned in Chapter 5. Using biofeedback, I can energetically test for a negative pattern a person continues to repeat throughout life. One example would be a pattern of "Judgement," which means the person continually judges himself and others, or a pattern of being a "Victim," which indicates the person experiences injustices and blame. I chose a nice lady whom I felt had good energy. I hoped she was my saving grace. I read her pattern as "Relationships," which means she would struggle in relationships. She refuted that this wasn't the case and said my reading did not make sense.

To the audience I now appeared completely incompetent. My tolerance to humiliation had already reached its peak halfway into the demonstration. My mind went blank and other blunders followed. I felt I was in a big black hole with no way out.

Can someone pleeeeease call the stage manager? I need to know where the secret trap door is located — ASAP!

For my healing career, it felt like the biggest disaster since the sinking of the Titanic.

My friends and peers had concerned looks on their faces and questioned why it all went so wrong. Some of the audience members left early and some later said there was bad energy in the room. Clients cancelled their healing appointments after witnessing my presentation. Hardly any students committed to my training courses and my reputation was in jeopardy.

After the event, I analysed everything that had happened. Seeds of doubt were planted in my mind about my healing abilities, but intuitively I sensed this had a greater meaning and better outcomes would follow. I was not going to waste the messages or the lessons the event was teaching me.

Despite that fateful day, the following week I was scheduled to present in a different state in Australia. I had some trepidation that the same results might happen, but I was ready, armed and dangerous, as I used my Forensic Analysis to make sense of the negativity that occurred in my hometown. I proceeded to make the right changes, and turn the pain into my power. I removed the negative energy directed at me from some of my peers who had once taught me along my healing journey. They did not like the success or attention I had been getting. To my relief, the next event proceeded effortlessly and some amazing transformations took place.

That devastating day became an important teaching tool to improve my healing abilities and the standard of my healing presentations. I realised how powerfully the people I associated with affected outcomes in my personal and business life.

The effect of other people's emotions and intentions (which is all energy) is intensified as society makes a shift to acknowledge and respond to feelings and emotions. Therefore, *other people's energy and emotions are affecting and impacting us on a greater scale than ever before.* The energy of everything has become more tangible.

There is a distinct shift in old values and beliefs that are no longer serving the human race. These range from competing or fighting with one another, to seeking cooperation and harmony. There is a shift from the old thinking — that we are separate from each other — to the notion we are all *connected* and one.

The old belief, that we have no power or choice in the way we live our lives, is being replaced by a new awareness that we are co-creators of something big and meaningful. Showing love and respect for each other, the Earth, and ourselves is paramount to moving into a brighter future. The energy of our emotional bonds to the relationships in our lives will either help or hinder our success in more ways than we acknowledge.

THE POWER OF RELATIONSHIPS

The secret to powerfully moving forward is to analyse all of your past and present relationships. All your relationships consist of the emotions you generate and the emotions of others who are connected to you. Emotions are the most POWERFUL source of energy, as you are an energetic being. You have an energy field that holds everything you are.

Your energy field contains emotions that are continually emitting a vibration to attract similar people and situations. When you know what is in your energy field, then you know why you attract your situations. Furthermore, you have the power to *control* what goes in and out of your energy field by choosing your relationships. When you take responsibility for your own choices and the people and situations you connect with, you control what you attract and change your success levels!

WHAT'S YOUR CURRENT "ENERGY STATUS"?

Your current "energy status" consists of the accumulation of your past and present relationships and circumstances. Negative relationships embed negative imprints and accumulate in your energy field unless they are addressed and removed. These imprints create life blocks, bad luck, detrimental relationships, financial losses, pain, stress, and most health issues. Negative relationships leave a negative residue that grows like cancer. Everything begins with energy, so choosing better energy changes the unwanted situations you have been attracting.

Your close relationships have the most impact on you as they build stronger cords and connections. The energy of the relationship builds over time with feelings, conversations, anniversaries, memories; an "energetic imprint" builds on each connection you have with another person. Therefore, if your longstanding connections are negative, it takes longer to undo the harm and negative impact they cause.

Analysing your relationships more thoroughly will show you how they affect your life. You may think your relationships are harmless and have no relevance in your life. *Life is a science,* which is great to know if you know the scientific formula. If you want more in life then you need to change your relationships with the people connected to you, and remove old ties. People who desire change in their own lives will want the same for you. Those who resist change for themselves will put the same resistant energy on you.

YOU ARE LIKE A MAGNET

Emotions attach to you that match the vibrational frequency of your feelings and emotions. The following table categorises the negative vibrations and positive vibrations that attract each other.

List 1 shows the negative vibrations that can hold similar frequencies to each other. The first ten vibrations listed are the most damaging. List 2 shows the positive vibrations that hold the most healing and constructive outcomes, the top ten being the most powerful.

LIST 1 – Negative	LIST 2 – Positive
Hate	Love
Anger	Self-worth
Jealousy	Gratitude
Blame	Compassion
Fear	Respect
Negativity	Empowerment
Ungratefulness	Integrity
Disrespect	Responsibility
Insincerity	Freedom
Control/Manipulation	Connectedness
Low self-worth	Safety
Shame	Wholeness
Deceit	Patience
Hurt	Openness
Victimisation	Happiness
Guilt	Encouragement
Impatience	Stability
Rigidity	Generosity
Depression	Transparency
Disconnected	Positivity
Unstable	Balance
Greed	Strength
Hidden agenda	Sincerity
Disempowerment	Peacefulness
Weakness	Honesty

As like attracts like, the aim is for you to create and connect to the positive emotions. The more positive vibrations you feel, and the people around you feel, the more positive energy you will accumulate to attract more of the same.

MAKE CONSTRUCTIVE CHOICES

One lesson that came from my "Titanic" presentation was how the beliefs and biases of others physically present or energetically affected my outcomes. If someone has a predetermined idea or belief of what an outcome should be, they will affect the outcome of what they are observing. If many people share the same belief, the energy of their belief is magnified, affecting the outcome in an even more powerful manner. You are affected by the beliefs of the people you surround yourself with. If a person does not have the belief that she can accomplish something, she usually won't have the belief that you can. This is all done on an unconscious level. It is an energetic exchange that takes place every minute you are around someone. The more time spent with a person, the greater that person can affect your circumstances, for better or worse.

"We don't see things as they are, we see them as we are."
Anaïs Nin

Lynne McTaggart's book *The Field* supports this theory when she refers to the Observer Effect Experiment, when quantum physicists demonstrated the "observer's bias," or how the beliefs about an experiment affect the outcome. They showed how an experiment with atoms was altered when the scientists observed the experiment with an expectation of what the outcome would be. This was demonstrated to have altered the outcome when it was compared to the controlled experiment with no observers.

McTaggart states, "To think is to affect." She says that discoveries in quantum physics are indicating that everything is connected: "At one time, we believed there was one system of 'large' physics, and another system of physics the 'small'. We're now understanding that there is only one system of physics — the laws of the quantum world which are applicable to the world at large, the great big world of visible matter. Those laws suggest that the observer has an effect on reality. And there is evidence that our thoughts have the capacity to change physical matter. That being the case, we have to rethink almost everything, because we've perceived a world based on separation, but the world that we're discovering now is a world of unity.

I can now see how the "observer's effect" changed the outcomes in my demonstration. I have since realised the best demonstrations occur when there is a group of people who have a positive belief in my abilities.

This concept also applies to your personal and business lives. People who have no belief in themselves will energetically keep you at their level unconsciously. The people who have positive and unlimited beliefs about themselves will project the same beliefs on you.

I believe that you cannot find something in someone else unless you find it in yourself first.

SCIENCE PROVES EMOTIONS CREATE OUTCOMES

Science has proven that negative emotions reduce the function of the immune system. In the 1980s, Dr David McClellan conducted an experiment during which students watched a video of Mother Teresa helping the poor while he simultaneously measured their IGA levels (IGA refers to Immunoglobulin A, a chief antibody in the human body). Dr McClellan found the students had a rise in IGA levels when they watched the video, as it aroused the emotions of care and compassion associated with Mother Teresa.

In 1995, Rein, Atkinson and McCraty conducted a study, "The Physiological and Psychological Effects of Compassion and Anger." A group of students purposefully created and focused on feelings of anger and their IGA levels dropped to half of what they had originally been, suppressing the immune system. Even after six hours, the levels had still not returned to normal. The study also showed that positive and compassionate emotions influence the immune system for up to six hours.

DNA PHANTOM EFFECT EXPERIMENT

In Chapter 5, I mentioned David Wilcock's book *The Source Field Connection*, which made a reference to the DNA phantom effect experiment where photons in a container stay in the same pattern as the DNA when the DNA strand is removed. From this we may conclude that our DNA leaves an imprint and attracts particles to it that become a physical form. As I mentioned earlier, we leave a trail of ourselves everywhere we go, which would explain why places and objects could arouse certain emotions and feelings in us.

Further explanation of this phenomenon in Wilcock's book shows that people with the most coherent brainwaves (feeling love) and incoherent brainwaves (anger) have a strong effect on changing the DNA. This experiment was conducted by Dr Glen Rein, who revealed that DNA behaves in direct response to human consciousness. DNA unwinds when a cell is about to divide or has been damaged, and it winds back again when it is working to repair and heal itself.

Are you now realising the amount of power others have over you and how much your own thoughts and feelings affect your own life and others?

REMOVE WEAK LINKS

The people who are connected with you are your building blocks in life. Just as a chain has no strength if one link is broken, the same can be said about your life. When there is a situation or person in your life who is negative, that one person can undo all your hard work or affect you in ways that you have never considered.

Weak links are people who are toxic to your life or have hidden agendas. These people can drain your energy, so create boundaries and expectations with the people you allow into your life. Weak links can be found anywhere in your life, whether it be on Facebook, Twitter, your phone, at work, among your friends or family, or your neighbourhood. It is time to clean out the weak links in your life so you can build a life on support and empowerment.

NEGATIVE EMOTIONS

Negative emotions and vibrations include feeling guilty and being manipulated by another person. Feeling responsible for someone else's emotions when they are capable of managing themselves allows you to be blamed for their life. For instance, you might be offered a new overseas job and you decline the position because you feel guilty knowing your mother will miss you. If you accept the job, your mother can manipulate you from afar. You feel guilt when she directs the responsibility of her happiness onto you, and this builds negative emotions and energy. This can turn into bad luck so the job doesn't work out and you have to come home, back to your old neighbourhood, back to Mama.

This can also work in reverse: children can manipulate and place guilt on a parent. We have all met those kids at one time or another (not yours of course!).

They say jealousy is a curse and I have reversed many curses that came from other people's jealousy. Jealous people unintentionally (or even intentionally) wish harm on another person whose success or happiness the jealous person resents. I have witnessed shocking outcomes from other people's feelings of jealousy in my own life and the lives of my clients. One client example was with a young girl whose aunt was jealous of her because she was very pretty and her own daughter was plain looking. The aunt directed so much jealousy onto the girl that her lovely long hair began to fall out and left a bald patch on her head. The doctors couldn't find a reason for her condition. When the curse was removed, all her hair grew back.

Resentment and anger are negative emotions. When these emotions are directed to you they can act as a magnet for other negative energies. This often leads to conditions such as chronic pain, back problems, financial problems, skin conditions, and more. People become resentful for many reasons. One result of this can be a compulsion to self-sacrifice, or put yourself last.

Do you remember your mother ever saying, "All the things I've done for you and look what I get!" When you put yourself last on the to-do list then you will always feel empty inside, and need something to fill you up, so you seek it from others. This common sacrifice pattern causes resentment, unhappiness, and an unfulfilled life. It allows your happiness to be dictated by others.

ALWAYS TRYING TO DO THE RIGHT THING?

I once commented to the mother of a daughter I was working with that the mother needed to be more particular about the people she allowed into her life. She responded that she attempts to do the *right* thing, be non-judgmental, and accept people for who they are. I replied that she could not be more wrong, as her beliefs and behaviour were costing her.

The mother had brought her daughter to see me about a chronic illness. I finally got to the bottom of the illness by using my investigative process of who, what, when and why scan lists so the specifics can be identified around an issue and the answers confirmed. The illness was triggered when the mother's angry sister was present at a family occasion. The mother described her sister as, "angry, jealous, and competitive." Just as unhealthy or toxic foods will destroy your health, the same can be said for toxic and unhealthy people when they transfer their negative energy on you.

THE POWER OF EMOTIONAL STATES

People underestimate the power of emotion and what it can do to a person. Love can heal a person and hate can embed a curse. You can go for years and not realise how the people around you — or the people from your past — have affected outcomes in your life. Your energy field becomes so chaotic, clouded, and filled with negativity that you cannot see the forest for the trees. Your senses are dulled to what is really happening around you.

I have learned this lesson due to the pain I have endured by not being "awake" enough to realise what had been going on around me. I was overly concerned about making sure the people around me were happy, so I ignored my own gut feeling and messages.

Even though you think your friends want the best for you, I have written a checklist (Positive Energy Index, or PEI) so you, too, can read between the lines to see if you are a good friend to others and if you have good, genuine friends around you. It takes a person who is genuinely balanced or a person who truly understands universal laws to be aware of her influence on others and the influence others have on her.

People who "pretend" in life and don't reveal who they really are, have unresolved anger and target this negative emotion on the people around them. I have met many people who appear to be nice, sweet, and happy, but who were only pretending. These people have opened my eyes to what underlying inadequacies can do to the people in one's life, and the detrimental effects they have on finances, health, and relationships. The way to really judge a person's sincerity and motives is to look at what he or she says about others, how he or she treats others, and how you feel when you are with them. Of course, how they treat you or speak to you needs to be considered.

I now recognise that almost every health condition or life situation begins with negative emotions towards ourselves, others, the universe (the Source, or God) and other people's negative emotions towards us. I will be using the word "Source" as a generic term. You can substitute the word of your choice such as Universe, God, life force, etc.

FREEING WOMEN EXERCISE:
POSITIVE ENERGY INDEX (PEI)

STEP 19: RELATIONSHIPS ASSESSMENT; WHERE YOUR POWER IS SOURCED!

Create a list of your closest relationships. In the next step we will reveal the PEI rating for each person which may be revealing.

STEP 20: DISCOVER YOUR POSITIVE ENERGY INDEX (PEI)

A) For each person in your current circle, consider the following description of traits and tendencies. Assign a rating for each person for each negative category listed below. *The rating should be between 1 and 10, with 1 being the most accurate description and 10 the least accurate description.*

Dog ear or bookmark this page. You should use the PEI for all your relationships into the future.

JUDGMENTAL: (1 being most accurate, 10 least accurate)

They make derogatory comments about others in general. They persuade you to not like someone. They use a "grooming" process to disempower others so they can have power over them. They make some positive comments, and then negate them with derogatory comments. They speak negatively about others, or they hide their true negative feelings about others.

JEALOUS: (1 being most accurate, 10 least accurate).

They are competitive or jealous of others' achievements. They refrain from expressing genuine happiness for others' success. They lack self-worth and attempt to appear "better" than others. They complain about others' income, integrity, or community status. They are unsuccessful in their life plans and relationships.

BLAMING: (1 being most accurate, 10 least accurate)

These people blame others when things go wrong. They make comments such as, "They did this to me and it was wrong." They play the victim or martyr role. They complain about types of service they receive or a product they bought.

MANIPULATIVE: (1 being most accurate, 10 least accurate)

They use subtle negative comments about others, and then talk about their own achievements. They describe how great others say they are. They claim to be better than others so they appear to have authority. They lie and exaggerate the facts and enjoy gossip. They pursue arguments and make threats to others. They choose litigation as a process to get what they want.

ANGRY: (1 being most accurate, 10 least accurate)

These people have unresolved anger towards others. They hold suppressed and unresolved emotions from childhood. They are justice fighters who fight other's battles for those they think are treated unfairly. They want others to change to their way of thinking or beliefs. They hide who they really are. Their anger seeps out in different settings, for instance while driving, watching TV, or speaking about others.

FAKE: (1 being most accurate, 10 least accurate).

These people pretend they are something they are not, they do not know their true identity or what they really like. They're secretive and hide their true intentions. They have ulterior motives, and seek ways to take advantage of you. They are convincing in covering up their true feelings, they lie quickly and easily. They are insincere in their compliments. They make deliberate acts to show they are trustworthy, and then abuse their trust. When confronted, they deny any wrongdoing, and blame others.

BAD RELATIONSHIPS: (1 being most accurate, 10 least accurate).

This group includes anyone who has negative and toxic associations with others, especially family members and friends. They are vengeful and hold grudges.

LOW SELF-WORTH: (1 being most accurate, 10 least accurate).

These are chronic apologisers who have hazy boundaries and can't say no. They are indecisive, afraid, and ashamed of exposing their true selves. They deflect praise and suspect compliments are insincere. They regret their past and give in easily.

They predict their own failure, and set low targets for themselves.

DISCONNECTED: (1 being most accurate, 10 least accurate).

These people are unaware of their own behaviour and the feelings of others. They live in fear and will experience constant overwhelm. They struggle in trusting their life will work out. They feel stressed by life, are unreliable, and lack real empathy for others. They feel as though the world is distorted or not real (derealisation). They experience memory problems that aren't linked to physical injury or medical conditions.

HOW BAD DO THEY FEEL? (1 being most accurate, 10 least accurate).

How does this person "feel" to you? Do you feel drained and unhappy, or do negative things occur after you connect with this person? Do you act negatively around this person when you are normally positive? Do you hesitate spending time with this person?

Calculate PEI Rating:

B) Find the PEI (Positive Energy Index) by rating a person for each of the categories above, then add the total and divide it by 10 = PEI.

Example: 62 (Total) / (Divide) 10 = 6.2
Check rating of 6.2 placed in the index.

C) Reviewing the Positive Energy Index Rating Guide
In our example, 6.2 score suggests the person in your relationship is "Reliable and good company". The higher the score confirms you're onto a good thing. Below a score of 5 may reveal some unwanted news of the negativity this person brings into your life.

PEI RATING

10: Awesome. You have struck gold-hang on tight to this person!

8-9: Genuine, positive and supportive–great person.

6-7: Reliable and good company.

5: Sitting on the fence-the jury is still out.

3-4: Not looking healthy at all-highly toxic.

1-2: Bad-run for hills and don't look back!

Use the PEI method for each person in your current circle into the future.

RESOURCE:

Positive Energy Index PEI online rating form is free at http://marisarusso.com/fug-reader/

YOUR SOURCE OF POWER

People who give you the most joy in life are the people who unconditionally love you for who you are. People with whom you relate to, often have similar qualities to yourself. You will become the "average" score of the people around you. Each time you associate with someone, it impacts your energy field. It is paramount to have a network of people who support and accept you for who you are.

Intentionally seek to create relationships with people who offer genuine relationships. Good relationships give you emotional support, which is like gaining more energy or power. *The best people to surround yourself with are those who are emotionally balanced and take responsibility for their outcomes.*

STEP 21: YOUR PERSONAL POWER NETWORK

List ten people in your new supportive network you will seek out

The list will contain people you know who have the qualities and attributes that will support you. Intentionally choose these people to create relationships. They may be on your outer circle right now so run the numbers and use the PEI to assess compatibility.

These exercises will train you to think more clearly about the impact you have on others, and the impact others have on you. In my experience, *emotion is the most powerful form of energy.* You can now use it to your advantage and be more intentional in your creations.

The more connected you become, the more you feel and the more you will intuitively know, and words will not be needed. When words are spoken to you, you will be able to discern their integrity. This process opens you to becoming more sensitive; however, this does not mean that you have to lose your power or play small. This means you can be both: sensitive to energy *and* powerful!

CHAPTER 8:
EXPRESSION

"Little girls should be seen and not heard," my father scolded, keeping his voice low enough so that the rest of the party could not hear.

My uncle was having his eighteenth birthday party at my grandfather's home, and we were invited to enjoy the celebrations. My mother's father, was a very kind man who treated me well and I felt safe and secure in his home. I was eight years old when I wandered into the party room, staring at the "grown-ups" who were talking loudly to each other. It seemed unusual to me, because I hadn't witnessed people enjoying each other's company and having loud conversations like this before — especially in my home. I was more accustomed to commands, criticisms, yelling, and intimidations: "Do what I say or else!" type of conversations. I was not allowed to respond, so the conversation was limited to receiving orders — it was never a dialogue.

I stood amongst the adults looking up in amazement. Without thinking, I blurted out, "What's everyone talking about?"

The room grew silent as all eyes turned towards me. A couple of people burst out laughing, but it was not funny for me, as my father quickly dragged me to the drinks room. He ordered me to sit in the corner for the remainder of the evening to repent. I felt so embarrassed about what I had said, and hoped no one would see me for the rest of the night. I thought I was a disgrace to society as I sat there alone.

I was always very timid about speaking in public. I guess I can thank my father for the way my face would turn beetroot red if I was asked a question or needed to speak up in a group setting as I got older. Even worse, when I felt myself blushing, I became more embarrassed and went even redder. I radiated so much heat from my embarrassment that I looked like I had a chronic case of sunburn.

SO WOMEN HAVE TO BE SILENT?

So who made the rule, "Little girls should be seen and not heard"? I know that I am not the only female who was forced to abide by it. I want to see the rulebook where it is written and I want a conversation with the author!

Fortunately, I no longer blush or feel embarrassed when expressing myself. I have peeled away the layers of filters and conditioning that made me someone I was not. What now remains is my true self. No more feeling embarrassed that what I have to say is worthless or not valued. My message is important. I want to give women the permission they have been denied to lead, speak, and be great! In less articulate words, *go kick ass* and don't let the voices from your past stop you from doing what you were born to do.

I believe that the following Bible scripture (there are many others) may reveal where the conditioning and beliefs about women speaking out come from:

1 TIMOTHY 2:11-12: "A woman should learn in quietness and full submission. I do not permit a woman to teach or to assume authority over a man; she must be quiet."

The repercussions of these scriptures are evident everywhere. I see signs in every corner of the globe that show how the scriptures are enforced. Even in Western "free-thinking countries" the statistics give evidence of women holding back when speaking.

One new study was conducted by scholars at Brigham Young University (BYU) and Princeton, and published by the top academic journal in political science, *American Political Science Review*. The researchers found that when a group of men and women meet to solve a problem, women speak less than men, by about 75%.

"Women have something unique and important to add to the group, and that's being lost at least under some circumstances," said Dr Chris F. Karpowitz, the lead study author and a political scientist at BYU.

When the group was asked to make a decision by unanimous vote, interestingly, things changed. When the focus was on building consensus, women were more likely to come forward with their thoughts and ideas, even when men outnumbered them.

Professor Tali Mendelberg of Princeton co-authored the study and confirmed the findings were consistent with a number of different situations:

"In school boards, governing boards of organisations and firms, and legislative committees, women are often in the minority and the group uses majority rule to make its decisions.

These settings will produce a dramatic inequality in women's floor time and in many other ways. Women are less likely to be viewed and to view themselves as influential in the group and feel that their 'voice is heard."

For their experiments, Karpowitz and Mendelberg formed 94 groups of five or more people. They asked them to decide the best way to split a sum of money earned by a group of people for completing a theoretical task. The groups discussed the issue for an average of 25 minutes. Some voted by secret ballot, and they decided either by majority or by unanimous vote.

They uncovered that when women were more involved, they affected the group's position in a way that resulted in more generosity being extended to the lower levels of the group.

"When women participated more, they brought unique and helpful perspectives to the issue under discussion," Karpowitz said. "We're not just losing the voice of someone who would say the same things as everybody else in the conversation." When the women outnumbered men, they felt less restricted and more open to participate and respond.

TOP TEN LIST OF WOMEN'S FEARS

Sheryl Sandberg, author of Lean In, started a social media campaign asking women, "What would you do if you weren't afraid?" The responses clearly showed what holds women back from taking leadership roles. Here's the summary of the top ten responses:

1. **Claiming Success**

   Women have been conditioned to praise others, not to boast — and are often scorned for speaking openly about their accomplishments. This leaves the impression that male accomplishments are more important, leaving them feeling intimidated and reluctant to stand up and take credit where it is deserved. This can cause women to decline leadership roles.

2. **Everyday Sexism**

   Women are so accustomed to dealing with sexist remarks and attitudes that it has become the norm for most work places.

3. **Standing Up for Themselves**

   When boys stand up for themselves, they are applauded. When girls do it, they're often told they are too "bossy." As adults, we can compare this to the men in the office who "get the job done" and are respected. A woman with a similar style is often referred to as a "bitch."

4. **Following Their Dreams**

   Changing careers is scary for everyone, but it's riskier for women. There can be a lack of support for women with families, and pressure to stay inside traditional gender roles. Then there is the lack of pay equality to contend with, and the glass ceiling.

5. **Speaking Up**

   In *Lean In*, Sheryl Sandberg says, "I still face situations that I fear are beyond my capabilities. I still have days when I feel like a fraud. And I still sometimes find myself spoken over and discounted while men sitting next to me are not. But now I know how to take a deep breath and keep my hand up. I have learned to sit at the table."

6. **Looking the Way They Want To**

In the age of Photoshop, it's almost the norm for women to feel like their normal, healthy bodies are not acceptable.

7. **Travelling Alone**

It's a sad reality that there is a prevalence of violence against women that they don't feel safe travelling alone — especially at night. The ability to move about safely in peace and solitude is something all women deserve.

8. **Pissing People Off**

Young girls are praised for pleasing others, and are criticised for speaking up. This leads to a great deal of discomfort for some women when it's appropriate to express anger or ideas that will make others angry. Women don't want to be viewed as aggressive or opinionated.

9. **Being Judged**

Another problem women have is being conditioned to be people-pleasers, and they view their choices and assess options through the filter of public opinion. Whether it's their clothes, friends, or choices, women worry about being judged which has a limiting effect on their perceived choices.

10. Failure

The fear of failure is something everyone has to learn to deal with, but for women there are attitudes and mechanisms that really make success harder to attain. Women with a desire to accomplish something are sometimes deterred by the worry of being ashamed of failing at it.

Women need to come to terms with the possibility of failure, and realise that it's okay.

Take the lead from Sheryl Sandberg and let's bring balance back into our homes, workplaces and global leadership.

FREEING WOMEN EXERCISE:
CONVERSATION AND EXPRESSION ANALYSIS

If you have ever engaged in a conversation that was one-sided or you didn't have the confidence to reply in the manner you wanted, ponder different ways you could have responded after you leave the situation. Practise articulating the exact words so you are familiarising yourself with responding in a confident, calm manner next time a similar conversation arises. You can practise when you are alone, driving in your car, or taking a shower. Speak to them out loud so the responses become natural for you.

This process of expressing yourself takes time to learn. It builds your confidence and feelings of self-worth. When you respond in an empowered, assertive manner, you will get more of what you want, and less of what you don't want, without feeling guilty or frustrated. Learning to respond in this manner will help you to avoid acting or speaking out of anger, and then feeling guilty for your actions. Remember, your feelings do matter, and what you have to say matters!

STEP 22: Switch the Conversation

Examine relationships/situations in which you refrain from expressing your opinion.

If you analyse your patterns, you will see that you do the same dances with the same people. They say the same old things and you respond in the same old ways. In other words, they waltz and you waltz. But now when they waltz, you must do the cha-cha. You are going to respond differently; however, you need to learn the cha-cha so you are prepared. Time to practise new dance steps!

Examples:

1. Your partner responds that you are too sensitive and over-reacting when you express that you feel criticised.
2. Your mother ignores your frustrations that she gives preferential treatment to your brother.
3. An ungrateful colleague asks you to do more work when you are already over-loaded with work.
4. Your father is critical of your career choices and leaves you feeling judged.
5. Your boss is judgmental and intimidates you.

Make a list in your journal of some recent conversations that are unresolved:

EMPOWERED RESPONSES

Practising an empowered response prepares you for the situation when it arises. It also sends the message to the receiver energetically so they receive it on an unconscious level.

Practise assertiveness; Talk in an assertive manner in front of a mirror or with a friend. Pay attention to your body language, ensuring it shows confidence to match your words.

Practising this new way to respond prepares you for the situations that arise when you feel hurt, angry, disempowered, or you bite your tongue and say nothing. It takes practice to respond in a calm, assertive manner. It is necessary to respond in a manner that expresses how you feel; otherwise your hurt feelings and anger mount up until you blow your stack!

In my healing practice, the most common complaint I receive from women is that they feel frustrated by their partner's behaviour, and they feel too intimidated to express themselves. They feel their relationships are a one-way ticket: they give and their partners take. When I address their male partners in a therapy session, there is a common thread of thinking. They don't perceive they have any issues in their relationship. Men seem to think it is a woman's role to endure discomfort and ignore her feelings, and as long as their (men's) needs are met, everything is fine. Men even admit they invalidate their partner's feelings by accusing them of being "too sensitive" or "over-reacting."

THE HANDBALL

The word "handball" comes from Australian football rules. It is used when a football player makes a fist and hits the ball to their team members to pass it to them, as throwing is not allowed.

In this situation, use the handball rule, and send unwanted comments back to where they came from! If they are negative, disempowering or unflattering — relay the comments back to the person who said them. For example, suppose your partner blames you because his computer crashed, when you used it the day before. You handball back what he said: "Are you blaming me for your computer not working because I used it yesterday, when you have been working on it for the last four hours?" Require them take responsibility for what they have said.

STEP 23: CONVERSATION ROLE PLAY

Your new response to the situations you listed in Step 22:

Example:

Other Person: "You're just too sensitive!"

You: "I feel my needs are invalidated when you tell me I am over-reacting. If you want this relationship to work, I would appreciate you refrain from belittling me in front of your friends and validate my needs and feelings."

Refer to your journal and write new, empowered responses to the unfinished conversations that are still playing out in your mind. Now practise them out loud. For extra credit, practise with a friend.

BECOME A NEGOTIATOR AND INFLUENCER

It can be confusing to learn how to negotiate your relationships or learn when enough is enough. What do you do when you are stuck in a bad marriage or relationship? How do you remove the guilt and shame others direct on you if you don't comply with their requests? Many women are suppressed and lack the ability to express their needs in an empowering manner. Many women keep silent and "soldier on" just as I had been doing. I have experienced all these relationship scenarios and they never lead to a happy or healthy life. Still, there are people in your life who will always be there, either by choice or by circumstance. You'll need to learn how to negotiate conversations, ask for what you need, and return the balance of power.

This journey to reconnect and empower yourself will require an action plan to create equal and harmonious relationships. You will learn how to determine if a relationship is worth continuing, and how to remove the angst of ending a relationship. There are formulas and action plans to keep you in control of your relationships and to maintain them in a positive and healthy state. This opens the door to experiencing fulfilling and loving relationships. Living with supportive, loving relationships makes this often-difficult journey worthwhile.

CHAPTER 9:
GRATITUDE

Uluru, the big red rock in the centre of Australia, is known for its magical healing powers and spiritual ambience. Some years ago, I did some research into the amazing energies of Uluru and spent eight days conducting healing work amongst the indigenous Anangu people. I had the crazy intention of meeting a witch doctor so I could expand my knowledge in the Forensic Healing course I had been writing. When I arrived, to my surprise, I learned the Aborigines were an insular race, and it took some persuasion to encourage them to be open to talk about their culture, their wisdom, and their deep respect for the planet.

We were given special permission to visit sacred sites and film in areas like the cultural centre. It was there that I found the "sorry book;" a compilation of letters from Uluru visitors who wrote about negative life experiences they encountered after removing rocks or red soil as souvenirs from Uluru. The park rangers reported they receive thousands of returned rocks, soil, and sorry letters every year. I was mesmerised by the stories in the "sorry book." Most of the letters explained the writer didn't originally believe in superstition or karma. Their opinions changed radically after they experienced family deaths, car accidents, bad relationships, and serious illnesses *en masse*. Here are some samples:

"I never believed it is true but now after two years I think it is. I made the biggest mistake of my life when I took some of the red sand. Since then a lot of bad things have happened to us ... I had my first miscarriage and then my father got lung cancer and died. I then had a second miscarriage and then an ectopic pregnancy. The doctors had to remove a tube to save me. The father of my closest friend died with cancer and my aunt died. I am still not pregnant..."

"I am a Christian and I was not superstitious when I took the red dirt ... since taking the dirt the same year my husband had prostate cancer, a heart attack and then died with rapid, progressive aphasia. My brother-in-law then died with brain cancer, my daughter-in-law lost her mother and my son-in-law lost his mother. My son is now diagnosed with pancreatic cancer. I now deeply regret what I have done..."

I was incredulous as I read letter after letter from the Uluru visitors describing their negative karmic experiences from disobeying the Aboriginal cultural law and removing the soil or rocks from Uluru. These stories and bad luck that followed from disrespecting a sacred place are representative of life and our planet. Karma does come back to bite people when they disrespect the planet and the human race. It is more evident that bad karma is intensified when a person disrespects or discredits someone or something that is deemed sacred, or a person living a divine purpose in making this world a better place. It seems the consequences are more serious.

I have seen many examples where very kind and loving people encounter people who disrespect them or treat them unfairly. The perpetrators ultimately experience the reality of negative karma.

IS KARMA A BITCH?

The following story I have never forgotten as it demonstrated just how real karma is.

Marika didn't have a mean bone in her body. She was a very kind Greek lady who came to see me for her emotional stresses. She was one of those sweet European women who just wanted the best for everyone. Marika had a loving husband, great kids, and everything was going well in her life except for her finances. She explained that she had been enjoying years of great financial success then suddenly, following a bad decision, her family lost all their assets. Things just went from bad to worse from that moment. When reading her energy field, I determined the cause came from a curse placed on her by her sister-in-law who harboured jealousy of her success. Marika then made an interesting statement; she said her sister-in-law had suffered financial losses after she did. Marika then started helping her sister-in-law by giving her what little money she had.

At the end of the healing session, Marika divulged a horrific experience of losing her unborn child. It happened many years ago when her body became swollen due to toxaemia. When she visited her doctor to explain her concerns, he curtly demanded that she stop fussing and sent her home untreated. Marika obediently returned home; however, the pain became so intense it stressed the unborn baby, who began kicking insistently in her womb.

Her husband, feeling quite desperate, drove Marika to the hospital; the nurses rushed her to a hospital bed and rang the same doctor, who was by then at his home. The doctor curtly instructed the nurse to apply hot towels, prescribed her painkillers, growling that he would arrive in the morning to deliver her baby. The next morning the doctor arrived, performed a Caesarean, and delivered a dead baby. The baby had died from the toxaemia.

I sat there in shock as Marika recounted the story. I asked her how she felt towards the doctor when it happened. Sadly she looked down at the floor and said, "What could I do?"

She then explained that following the loss of her baby, the same doctor unexpectedly lost his daughter in the Chernobyl disaster, a catastrophic nuclear accident in Ukraine. Marika lost a child from toxicity due to the doctor's actions and then he, too, lost a child from toxicity in Chernobyl. She added that she never wished the doctor any harm. She knew that the law of karma was true as she shyly admitted bad karma turns on people who exploit her.

When we create loving and respectful relationships, we create positive energetic connections and good karma. Depending on your thoughts or actions, positive or negative energy and consequences are created. Every action has a consequence. When you demonstrate respect and appreciation, positive energy and good karma flows to you. For example, respecting the Earth and living in a way that reduces waste and toxic load helps everyone to live a healthier and cleaner life whether others witness your deeds or not.

When there is respect shown to the Earth and all living creatures, it creates an abundant environment with nutritious foods and clean air to keep us healthy and happy. This is good karma. We live in a holographic universe where our bodies, our energy, and the nature of the Earth are all undeniably connected. *What you do to others, you do to yourself.*

KINDNESS TO SELF

If you deny yourself love and respect, then the universe can't give you love or respect. For instance, if you feel unworthy of receiving, or you think your value comes from giving and helping others, then the universe, which operates on your thoughts and energy, responds to your vibration. It matches this frequency and gives you more ways to serve and give to others. This often results in resentful feelings — as you give too much of yourself, you can end up feeling unappreciated and taken for granted. This is another negative emotion that attracts more negativity. You may as well just give in and "LOVE" yourself crazy!

KARMA FOLLOWS YOU

Karma can be carried over from past lives or other incarnations, and this is why some people are born in particular places and conditions. Your body holds a cell memory of your past lives and you come into this life with the same cell memory, or vibration. For instance, you may experience people taking advantage of you in this life. This could indicate that either:

1. You took advantage of people in past lives; or
2. You had low self-worth in your past lives and people took advantage of you.

KARMA CLEARING

The key to creating good karma in this life is to understand and learn from the messages that show up in your life, such as blocks, obstacles, or just feeling things are against you. Once you have understood the messages, keep your heart open to acceptance, forgiveness, and love. I have encountered clients who experienced a strong sense that they are paying off bad karma from a past life. They comment, "I must have done something bad in a past life" as they struggle with issues in their current life. When I read their energy field, their notions are confirmed, as their energy shows karmic consequences are involved in their life struggles. The good news is there is a way to speed up clearing your karma, and the following story of how the Ho'oponopono method came about will give you some idea how to create good karma and remove bad karma.

THE POWER OF THOUGHT AND GOOD INTENTIONS

From 1983 to 1987, Dr Hew Len worked at the Hawaii State Hospital in the high-security ward for the criminally insane, where violence was a daily occurrence. The environment was so stressful and hostile there was a consistent turnover of staff. When Dr Len began his work at the hospital, he decided to conduct his therapy on the patients without being in direct contact with them. He would only review the patients' files, and work on his perceptions and thoughts of the patients without meeting them personally.

Dr Len's theory was that we create and attract everything and everyone around us, and we are responsible for all our own problems. He would ask himself, "What is going on in me that I am experiencing these problems?" In other words, he believed that our energy field or subconscious mind contains a vibration that creates and attracts our relationships, environment, finances, experiences, etc. – everything we experience, even events and people that are external to us. He believed we can change them by acknowledging we are the creator or attractor of them.

He would ask the Divinity (source/God/universe) to erase memories in his subconscious mind and, as he did this, the patients improved. He also used four statements now called The Ho'oponopono Cleaning Statements. Over time, as Dr Len continued to clear and erase the negativity via this method, many of the patients returned home. The ward eventually closed down, as there were no more inpatients to house.

Dr Len notes that a common problem with therapists is their belief is to save people, when they are here to clear the shared memories they have in common with their own clients or patients. What a powerful message, knowing you can change what you are attracting by *letting go of judgments and perceptions of people and situations.*

FREEING WOMEN EXERCISE:
KARMA CLEARING

STEP 24: CLEAR YOUR KARMA

A) Create positive habits.

Any time you can lend a helping hand or give a smile to someone, do so. Always send love and blessings when you can. Focus on the positive so that you attract more of the same. Create good karma and release negative thoughts and feelings towards people or situations. Imagine throwing the negative thoughts and feelings in an imaginary "fire bin" and visualise them burning.

B) Ask the universe to erase your memories and perceptions.

For every negative situation you encounter, take responsibility that you are the creator of it (I hear you, you so want to blame the other person — after all, that person is the perpetrator — but resist those urges). When a negative situation arises, neutralise it by using Dr Len's methods. Here are the four statements to clear negativity in any situation:

- I'm sorry
- Please forgive me
- I love you
- Thank you

Repeat the Ho'oponopono cleaning statements when you have negative thoughts and feelings about your relationships, finances, or life problems and you will experience more flow and love in your life.

THERE'S ALWAYS A BIGGER PICTURE

Not all bad or negative things happen as the result of negative karma. Often the bad situations are trying to change you so that you can evolve spiritually (which creates a happier life). There can be more than one reason that things happen, so the key is to find the reason.

Your soul is on a journey. Karmic situations in which you find yourself today are both your soul's mirror and travel guide. Karma can show you where you've been and where you might go to learn the lessons for this lifetime. Through understanding your unique destiny, you can adjust your actions to either change an ongoing situation or gain a new perspective.

UNDERSTANDING THE FIVE FUNCTIONS OF KARMA

I accidently (or not) came across Dr Mitchell E. Gibson while searching online for information on energy healing. He is a board-certified forensic psychiatrist, writer, artist, and spiritual teacher. Dr Gibson has a medical degree and has written some interesting books on his experience of being able to "see" on the other side of the veil.

His extraordinary knowledge has been the missing link for me to understand more about the "unseen world" and convert this knowledge into healing corrections in my Forensic Healing course. In Dr Gibson's literature he speaks about the five types of karma. The first is *Divine Karma,* which is given by the creator and cannot be changed. The second is *Planetary Karma,* which relates to the location where a person lives and often determines outside influences, opportunities, and things like health and safety. The third is *Archetypical Karma,* which is the overall design of a person — destiny, abilities, talents, personality, and character. Fourth is *Stewardship Karma,* which determines material possessions and diseases a person has in a lifetime, and the fifth is *Personal Karma,* which relates to the personal lifestyle choices they make. When a person makes bad choices it increases bad karma; and wise karmic choices increase good karma.

> *"If the only prayer you say in your life*
> *is 'thank you,' that would suffice."*
> — Meister Eckhart

RESEARCH SHOWS GRATITUDE HEIGHTENS QUALITY OF LIFE

Two psychologists — Dr Michael McCollough of the Southern Methodist University in Dallas, Texas and Dr Robert Emmons of the University of California at Davis — studied gratitude and how it affects people.

They assembled three groups of people. The first group was instructed to keep a journal about their lives without any instruction on what to focus on. The second group was instructed to record any unpleasant or negative situations that happened, and the third group was instructed to record a daily list of things for which they were grateful.

When the study was completed, the results showed that people who wrote a daily list on gratitude said they felt better and more optimistic. They reported feeling more alert, happy, determined, and achieved more in their day. Dr Emmons says, "To say we feel grateful is not to say that everything in our lives is necessarily great. It just means we are aware of our blessings." People who do this are happier, healthier, more resilient, and more creative.

INGRATITUDE HAS CONSEQUENCES

I was really excited to be finishing the final module of the Forensic Healing course, which is called the "Spirit" module. It contains the most profound healing pathways I have ever used. It sheds light on new healing secrets, and it activates spontaneous healing forces in a person when the healing is applied. I'd searched for many years to assemble information and then I intuitively received instruction on how to use it to create healing pathways or healing corrections. I was then very keen to try the new healing secrets on my clients to confirm their effectiveness.

The Forensic Healing course we created contains manuals and videos to make it easier for students to learn. It allows them to watch any step of the course in their own home, at their own pace. For the final module, I approached a colleague and client named Kylie to be the model for the video. I wanted to offer her free healing sessions as for many years she attempted to heal herself and had seen dozens of practitioners (including myself), to no avail. She wanted to move past an abusive childhood, a boyfriend who left her for another woman, and feeling stuck.

Out of necessity, Kylie had been living with her mother ever since the separation from her boyfriend. More than two years previously he had moved in with his new girlfriend, and Kylie was still angry with her, even now. She often repeated the fact that she hated the new girlfriend, and how she'd stolen her boyfriend. During this time, Kylie experienced a lot of bad luck and was always complaining that people were out to get her, and showed their dark side to her.

Kylie happily agreed to be the model when we filmed the process of the healing steps of the new "Spirit" module. When the new healing pathway was finished and filming was over, she commented that it was the first time in her life she had felt so peaceful, happy, and energised. It was a brand new experience for her and she seemed elated at the changes.

I then challenged her. I questioned what her new feelings for the ex-boyfriend's girlfriend were. I was hoping for a positive response as her life had changed so dramatically in that moment.

"I still hate her," was the immediate response.

This surprised me. Kylie was a trained psychologist, had completed dozens of healing courses, and was trained in Neuro-Linguistic Programming, which teaches you how to speak constructively, so you create and attract the things you want.

Barely seconds after she responded to my question, the entire healing began to reverse. Within five minutes, she complained she felt unwell. The following day she contacted me to blame me for the way she was feeling. At that moment, I realised how I had allowed her to complain and blame everyone else for her problems for years, and now she was directing her wrath at me.

The healing Kylie received was free of charge in exchange for modelling for the video footage and I was sincerely trying to help her. It appeared the universe decided she was ungrateful and reversed the healing with interest, leaving her feeling worse than when she came to see me. It was a learning moment for me to be more alert to people's unwillingness to change.

A grateful response could have been that she was thankful for the healing, and was ready to feel differently. I suggested a more positive approach could have been that she was choosing to forgive, but she continued to justify her position of hate.

THERE'S MORE SENSE IN LIFE THAN WE REALISE

Bad things happen to good people, and sometimes bad people get away with bad deeds. Where is the justice, and how can you believe in the law of attraction when some things seem so random and unfair? You can find the reasons that most things happen. I will admit there are some things that occur in the world that are hard to make sense of, and are definitely unfair and cruel.

My perspective on those unfathomable situations is that some people are so conditioned and closed down to their feelings, they are disconnected from the pain they inflict on others. However, for the majority of situations, I can clarify why people attract their circumstances. The answers have come from years of trying to answer the "why" questions and learning universal laws — understanding that all choices have consequences.

JUDGEMENT DAY

People talk about the day of reckoning or "Judgement Day." For most this can mean the coming of Christ, Armageddon, or the Mayan calendar ending. There is an ending and a new beginning, but not in the way people tend to think. I believe it is a time of new energy and new integrity being brought into the world. This is causing people to be held accountable for their actions, intentions, and thoughts, and their past is catching up to them. I believe the days of getting away with bad deeds and bad energy are over. Justice is being restored.

WORDS AREN'T NECESSARY

There is no more hiding who you are. The energy and consciousness in the world today has been raised, so that thoughts become things, intentions manifest, and beliefs are created. You are living in a world where you will be "judged" more fairly, as the world has become more transparent, intuitive, and more knowing. This is the lifetime where — providing you are living with integrity — you can truly access universal source energy and activate universal laws. You are living in a world where the energy of who you are will manifest the same types of situations and circumstances. Now you can really hold all the power to create what you want!

BREAKING FREE

For the "energy" inside you to change, you must move on from your past traumas and stresses. You need to resolve karma and relationship issues that have followed you for many lifetimes. The previous lifetimes (history) operated in a lower vibration with less integrity, which has ultimately caused a world of turmoil, pain, and stress, trapping people in their circumstances.

Since most of us want a different life and world, it seems our desires and requests for something better are causing the fast changes that are now occurring in the world. If you ever wondered why you are not achieving the outcomes you want, perhaps the following list will highlight the top ten reasons that can prevent you from progressing.

1. Hanging on to anger and resentment, versus letting go and choosing peace.

2. Blaming others for your situation. It is time to take responsibility and acknowledge that *you* are the attractor and creator of your life and circumstance.

3. Lacking gratitude, being judgmental, and living igno-rantly of universal laws, versus showing appreciation and acceptance, and educating yourself about universal laws.

4. Building bad karma (from this lifetime and past lifetimes), instead of building good karma and blessing others.

5. Thinking you are a victim, and choosing to give without receiving, versus making choices from an empowered state and knowing you are already worthy without proving it through giving.

6. Disrespecting yourself; allowing toxic people and substances into your surroundings or body, versus creating a cleansing and uplifting environment.

7. Acting negative, jealous, or opposing others who are successful and repeating bad stories or situations and gossip, instead of disciplining yourself to act in a positive manner, repeating positive stories and situations.

8. Not living your life purpose, being fake and pleasing others, versus following your feelings, passion, and desires and showing the world *who* you are.

9. Being controlling and not trusting the universe (continual worrying), instead of surrendering and demonstrating you can let go and trust that everything will work out.

10. Having low self-worth, ignoring your intuition and feelings, and not being in your integrity, versus loving yourself and following your intuition and feelings so you live in your integrity.

KARMIC BANK ACCOUNT

You are now living off the energy in your karmic bank account. Is your bank account filled with good karma or are you living "in the red" with bad karma? You have the power to build your bank account with good karma and energy, as the universe is responding to what you have accumulated. You now have the power to decide how your life plays out and your own personal energy field needs to be your priority.

SPRING CLEAN

Time for a spring clean! Choose a life plan that is fulfilling and energising so your bank account is full of the good stuff that manifests more of the same. Make a commitment that you are responsible for your feelings and creations. Take proactive steps that give you access to the powerful source of energy that is continually guiding you to the freedom and happiness you have been seeking.

CHAPTER 10:
BECOMING WHOLE

When it Hurts Enough, You Change

The last two years of my eighteen-year membership in the Mormon Church felt painfully uncomfortable. It was almost unbearable to attend church meetings. I would feel glaring eyes upon me, judging and condemning me as if I had done something wrong. The Mormons were a non-gambling people, so showing a poker face was not a practice they had learned, and their frowning faces said it all.

John's ex-wife and her family were working hard to discredit us within the church by fabricating stories about us. This was during the two-year court battle John's ex-wife initiated. At that stage I was married to John and we remained committed to the church even though we were not enjoying it. I started to see wide cracks in what I had once thought to be the only true church on the planet. After many happy years, my whole belief in the church was crumbling and so was my foundation. Things only got worse the longer we stayed.

We didn't have any extended family in the church. John's ex had a tribe of members born and raised there. They were all very strange people to say the least and they loved drama. Hence, things got really ugly. I stayed obedient to the church's teaching and "turned the other cheek," thinking my reward would be in heaven. I was left feeling sad and exhausted as I dreaded attending church meetings and Sunday worship. I thought I was being tested, and the experience was a trial of my faith.

After two long years of the ongoing saga, I began to have an intense dislike for Mormonism, yet I never thought I had the option to leave. I had given eighteen good years of service (not to mention 10% of our gross wages) to this church, yet I was bullied and ostracised. Looking back on it now, if they had a customer service guarantee policy, I would be asking for a full refund!

John had self-funded a two-year mission with the Mormons. I self-funded a five-month mission in Rome, which took every last Italian lira I owned. I was a great recruiter for the church and I was diligent about bringing in new business for them. As things progressed from bad to worse, I started to wonder why I would encourage anyone to join a church that was lacking so much integrity.

John was one to question everything. After practising meditation for some time he began to feel incongruent with his true feelings and being part of the church. When reviewing his New Year resolutions on the morning of 1st January 2006, he asked himself the ultimate question. "How would it feel to be without the church?" He felt a deep burden lift and renounced his membership in the church. This took me by surprise, and it planted a seed that I also had a choice. A couple of weeks later I attended a kinesiology workshop where I received a healing, and the therapist identified and removed the emotion of feeling guilty. The therapist didn't know any of my history and from that moment, I no longer felt obligated to return to the church. With relief in my heart, I too made the shift away from Mormonism.

Despite my decision, I still held a residual belief that the church was true. A few months later, while flipping through the TV channels, I came across a documentary on Joseph Smith, the founder of the Mormon Church. It objectively showed how Joseph Smith was a great storyteller and had an ambition of becoming the president of the USA. The documentary revealed many things about the church I had never questioned.

I had always been instructed to have faith and not to question the teachings or leaders. In fact, if you did question the leaders, you would be denied a temple recommend, which was a status symbol in the church. As I watched the documentary it awakened me to my gullibility and vulnerability. It left me feeling betrayed by the church as I realised I had believed in a lie. My belief system of the previous eighteen years was shattered.

Joining the church did however play a big part in saving my life when I was headed on a journey of self-destruction. When it was time to leave, it was hard for me to give up my loyalty. I had to experience enough negativity to cause me to leave. Back then, the signs needed to be dramatic, like a semi-trailer running me over, as I didn't know how to read messages from the universe. When I did finally leave the church, I found myself on a path much greater than I'd ever envisaged.

All the signs were saying to me to leave and not look back. I have since realised that when there are continual obstacles and negativity, that is a sign to take stock of what is going on. This is when you need to use your logic and gut feelings to make better decisions.

Now I acknowledge the signs, find the messages, and act on them. We are constantly being guided and constantly being answered. We just need to be awake and aware that the signs and answers are there. Now I pay closer attention to what I am guided to do, as I am "over" hardship and suffering. I am no longer stubborn in reading the signs to guide me to happiness and freedom.

Signs and messages show up more easily when you are asking for the answers to appear and you are open to receiving them. One of the signs that things are on track is when there is "flow and ease" in your efforts; this is a sign you are on the right path. I have also discovered blocks appearing when I am about to break through old patterns and move forward into better patterns. I can now distinguish more easily what messages I am getting and what I should do. Wouldn't it be nice to ask a question and get an answer?

GOOD SIGNS AND MESSAGES

I have enjoyed many discussions with the Aboriginals about the signs and symbolism they read from nature. During a visit to Uluru in Australia, we saw an amazing sign as we were driving to see the famous sunset at the big rock. We witnessed the biggest and most vividly colourful rainbow I had ever seen.

We stopped the car to take it in and embrace the energy of the moment. As we stood looking at the rainbow, I was aware of cars that drove past hurriedly to catch the sunset. The passing traffic missed the most amazing view. For me, a rainbow is a positive sign: a precursor to something amazing about to unfold. After it appeared, I was walking around one of the most sacred parts of Uluru, called the Kuniya Walk. As I turned the bend, there was Oprah Winfrey walking towards me!

What are the odds of meeting Oprah, one-on-one on a dirt trail in central Australia? John and I were alone on the tiny trail and Oprah was walking in front of her thirty-person film crew. She briefly stopped to acknowledge me (of course I was trying to suppress my manic excitement), and we exchanged a few words before being swamped by the media. Visiting with Oprah had always been on my vision board. It was like our deep respect for the land, the people, and helping them with healing had opened up the heavens to a miracle. It was a great learning experience for me.

FINDING ANSWERS

When you have unanswered questions about your life problems, or unresolved health issues, financial stresses, or relationship problems, there is a formula to find the answers. If you have searched everywhere to get answers to seemingly unsolvable conditions and could not find them, rest assured relief is in sight.

This information will allow you to take back your control, as you cannot leave answers to your problems entirely in someone else's hands. If you follow this process it will lead you to finding the answers for yourself, or lead you to the person who does have the answers. There is a reason and solution for everything. You just need to have the right mindset and look in the right places.

Since I have realised that following my intuition leads me to the right place at the right time, (even though at times it did not seem that way) my life is consistently guided to fulfilling relationships and endless possibilities. I have noticed that when there is an initial block in attempting to start something, such as a person's questionable behaviour, or things don't flow, these signs seem to be a message not to progress any further. If I push through the blocks, it usually leads to problems that could have been avoided and realising I'd ignored my initial feelings that were telling me not to take that particular path.

WHAT ARE YOUR BLOCKS TELLING YOU?

When something initially appears right and there is flow, this generally means that it is the right path to take, even if blocks appear along the way. Often the blocks are precursors to something positive and significant taking place. Hindsight is a wonderful learning tool as the people I have met during my healing career, the ones that initially felt right and positive, have endured the test of time and the relationships that showed problematic, have all ceased.

We are accountable for our choices. All choices have consequences. We have free will and more power over our life's journey than we give ourselves credit for. *Freedom and peace come from accessing this power.*

When you are spiritually aligned, aware and connected, you are led to be in the right place at the right time. You are led to the right information and prompted to follow your hunches or gut feelings. Your inner guidance system is a powerful system that gives you personal knowledge and wisdom. It needs to be accessed and used daily to *gain the maximum advantage in life.* I spent decades trying to remove the daily emotional and physical pain I endured. It took me years to find the answers to solve my problems against my doctor's diagnosis that I would have to live in pain forever. I am now pain-free. This seems remarkable when I look back at how hopeless everything once seemed.

Life consists of detective work, and constant change is necessary if you want to alter outcomes. If there is something in your life right now that is not working for you, then the answer is — you need to change. *What* to change is the million-dollar question! This final chapter will lead you to finding answers and solving problems faster than ever before.

The first thing to understand is Henry Ford's statement, "If you always do what you've always done, you'll always get what you've always got." And Einstein said, "One cannot alter a condition with the same mindset that created it in the first place."

Changing your mindset and actions will give you different results. If you apply the following eleven suggestions, you will shift your mindset and find solutions to daily questions or long-standing problems. It is true: if you ask, you will receive.

FINDING A BILLION-YEAR CONTRACT

I knew nothing about the Billion Year Scientology contract until I was searching for answers for three of my clients' bizarre and chronic conditions. These clients had very difficult conditions to solve. One client spent decades trying to resolve her chronic fatigue. Another endured years trying to leave an abusive relationship but kept returning. For six years, one mother had tried everything to relieve her child's extreme fears.

While I was searching for answers, I was led to the contract created by L. Ron Hubbard, the founder of The Church of Scientology and Dianetics. He designed a contract his employees, followers, and their children were coerced to sign. It contracted their souls and lives to the service of Scientology or the Sea Org (a unit of Scientology) for one billion years. This contract is still used today. If a follower does not fulfil the contract, he or she will endure hardship in every lifetime until the contract expires, after one billion years. It's like paying off a never-ending debt.

Dating from the 1950s, Scientology remains one of the most controversial religions today. Its cult-like following is a closed and secretive group subject to much interference from the church leadership, and this contract was created for Scientology to keep its power, decade after decade, lifetime after lifetime. Scientologists believe in reincarnation, so the contracted member is expected after death to return to Earth and serve as a Scientologist.

My Freeing Women Daily System ultimately led me to resolving my clients' dilemmas. I trusted that I would receive answers and enlightenment occurred while I was flicking on-demand talk and documentary media channels (seems to be one of my patterns of finding answers). I chanced (I hear you saying that nothing is by chance and you're right!) upon a woman talking about Scientology, who had signed a contract at age eight. I couldn't move close enough to the TV when she was speaking and I felt a compulsion to research all I could on the subject. When I found the information on the Scientology contract, I emailed one of my clients. As she was scanning through her emails and came to mine, she burst into tears. This was her message that there was truth in the information. When the reincarnated contract on her soul was released, her life was completely transformed and a fullness of energy returned to her.

BEING HELD HOSTAGE BY A CONTRACT

The three clients I mentioned previously had been contracted souls and, since being reincarnated, didn't know they were being held hostage by the contract. One of them even said she was living in a "cult like" family. When the billion-year contract is cancelled, people's lives change. Their negativity and anger leave, and their energy returns. Total transformations have been taking place with my clients and other Forensic Healing practitioners.

Read Your Messages:

The following list details some of the ways we can be shown messages:

- Numbers
- Animals/nature/ weather
- Flow/Block
- Feelings
- Media messages
- Patterns
- Dreams
- Songs
- Impressions
- Thoughts
- Books
- Your conversations, and other people's
- Radio
- Traffic
- Billboards
- Magazines
- TV talk and documentary channels
- Words
- Intuition
- Random events and situations
- Car number plates

I have continually asked myself the question, "What is my message?" This is usually the question I ask when things are not flowing, and the answers now come quickly and clearly as I have developed the confidence to now trust my answers. Over time, I have received confirmation I was accurate with my interpretations of the messages.

When I was religious, I never questioned anything as I was conditioned to believe that the Bible contained the answers to everything. Now I believe we have our own internal GPS that provides each one of us with answers and guidance to all things in our lives. Some of the answers don't always come in the time or way that you want. Sometimes I pause to "feel" my question as to why the answers are not coming to me — that's when I get a feeling I need to wait for certain things to take place first.

Knowing that you have this ability within you and are able to live this way is *true freedom*. Use it!

BEING SENSITIVE *DOES* GIVE YOU AN ADVANTAGE

My life has sometimes played out like a science fiction or fantasy novel that even I have found hard to believe. The unseen world of energy has become so tangible and undeniable that for most people, I seem a little too "alternative" or weird for their liking. My heightened sensitivity to feeling things has opened me to a new world that most people fear, resist, or deny. Even if I wanted to, it seems I don't have that option.

Using these strange abilities allowed me to find a resolution to a 45-year-old client who had a difficult relationship with her father for decades. She continually complained that he was negative, controlling, and antagonistic towards her. It was not until later we realised that in her teens her father found her on the kitchen floor close to death, after attempting suicide. In shock, he gave away a part of himself (a soul fragment) to save her. During the healing, when this soul fragment was returned to her father, the relationship changed completely. Her father's negative behaviour towards her suddenly ceased.

SYMPTOMS OF SOUL LOSS

When parts of your soul are missing, this can lead to depression, suicidal tendencies, anger, frustration, grief, addictions, insomnia, dissociation, anxiety, hopelessness, and loss of identity and purpose. Some obvious signs are when you say, "I've never been the same since…" or, "I felt like I lost part of me when…" You live your life never feeling whole, continually searching for something unknown, never realising your soul fragments have been given away, taken, or lost.

Shamanic healers can retrieve soul fragments, and can access the world of present and past lives. Acting on the idea that you can't heal what isn't there, the shaman journeys into the unseen world of energy to retrieve soul parts that are needed to make the person whole again. You can't reach your full potential or find your destiny if parts of your soul are missing. If you think your mission is to give to, care for, or love others, and you neglect your own needs in the process, you will deplete parts of yourself and eventually your soul. This can result in feeling resentful or empty, and cause you to fill your life with distractions, to fill the void in your heart and soul that you don't know you created.

The healthiest way to give to others is to first balance your own emotional, physical, and spiritual needs. Acknowledge and take care of your own needs before giving to others. This prevents burnout, and allows you to sustain the energy needed to give to others, and it won't matter if you receive anything in return or not. When you give from this place of balance, you naturally receive more than you give.

The healing process of making our souls whole is very important, as we have been fragmented from not only trauma and stress from this life, but also our past lives. Our souls are continually evolving and healing, and fragments need to be returned so that each person can reach his or her full potential and destiny. This lifetime is the opportunity for everyone to heal and reach the greatness they were always destined to live. *When your soul is whole, your life becomes whole.*

HEALING WORDS TO BECOME WHOLE

Words have power. Just as I use words to heal and return soul fragments, I have words to continue your healing journey.

The following words are to restore your worth, dignity, soul fragments, and love for yourself. Begin this process by taking deep breaths, knowing there is no other place you need to be. Imagine all the hurtful things that have been done to you are acknowledged and you hear the words:

I am sorry for what happened to you. I give back to you what was taken from you; I give it back with love, please forgive me for your suffering.

Imagine how it feels to release yourself from all the pain and hurt you have endured. Imagine your suffering lifted from your body, and white and gold streaming light cleans and dissolves the anger and resentment you have towards the people who

Imagine the freedom of being connected to the Earth and the energies of the blue sky vibrating through every cell of your body. Imagine your arms outstretched as you fall back on long, thick green grass that cushions you. Look up to that never-ending blue sky and feel the rays of the warm sun over your entire body. Feel the freedom and the peace that comes to you. Now allow the shamans to return your lost soul fragments to restore your soul to peace and calm.

Visualise the people who have supported you: those who have cared for and loved you, family, friends, children, or animals, now in your presence. Look at their faces and feel their love heal you, feel it fill your heart. Experience the power of what love can do and the power of healing that it has. Hear the message they have come to give you, which is, *"You are more than you could ever imagine. If only you knew how much you are loved."*

Thank them for their love and support. Now feel all the love you have ever given them. Now fill your heart with this love. Send this love to your heart and feel love for yourself. This is who you really are; this is who you are here to be. This is what you are meant to experience. *Now choose to be this love.* You are love.

Relax in this feeling and let it permeate your energy field as you live your life in this new feeling from this point forward.

Now I'm going to share the final step that will be part of your healing journey.

FREEING WOMEN EXERCISE:
DAILY SYSTEM

STEP 25: FREEING WOMEN DAILY SYSTEM

My goal with the Daily System is to give you a step by step process of the core principles and practises I have used to shift from a weakened, abused state to feeling like powerful creator in my life. I continue to live the Daily System every day to bring about constant change and an elevated state of being.

Start with your intention to solve one specific life problem. Add another as you solve, move forward. Practise the following system daily and keep a journal of messages and impressions that come to you until you feel you have your solution. The more you incorporate these steps into your life, the easier and faster your answers will come.

1. **Intention**
   Ask to be shown or led to information that will resolve your question or problem.
   Be clear and specific about the things you are seeking and note it down. Resist focusing on the problem or what you don't want. *Keep focused on what you do want.*

2. Trust and Surrender

Let go of control so you can be open to messages. If you control your life you won't trust the messages that are coming to you. The universe will prove you correct in your assumption that you cannot trust life (remember what Ford and Einstein said). Project a different message and let go of all control. Repeat the affirmation: "I choose to trust and surrender."

3. Listen

Ask for the answers to come, and then listen for the answers.

Listen to what others are saying or the stories they are telling, even if you think it has nothing to do with you. Your answers are staring you in the face. Take note of headlines and what shows up when you surf the Internet. You need to be alert, listen, take note and "feel" if the information is right for you. Messages can be confirmed through feelings, an inner knowing, your small voice within, or a peaceful feeling.

4. Feel

Stop and be still.

For every decision you make, practise feeling and asking yourself, "Does this feel right?" Make a habit of connecting to your inner guidance. Heighten your senses to the energy with which you surround yourself. Keep challenging and asking yourself, "How does this feel?" Then make choices that give you feelings of positivity, peace and calm.

5. **Open Mind**
Refrain from judgment and criticism, as you will only attract it back to you.
If your mind is limited, you will create a limited life. Believe that anything is possible and anything can be true. Most of our minds have been programmed to think in a limited manner. We are only now realising our true potential is much greater than what we are living. It's time to re-educate yourself to become your true unlimited self!

6. **Unwind Beliefs**
Question the source of your beliefs, as they become conscious thoughts.
Did your parents struggle in life? Did you have a religious upbringing based on guilt and fear? Do you believe yourself to be unworthy? Do you have limiting beliefs that hold you back? Do you believe you cannot be healed? If you have spent years searching for answers, you will need to erase this history and look at the problem with new eyes. Start with the basics — that is usually where the answers lie.

7. **Change Patterns**
Choose something new today.
Eat something different, take an alternate route, and call somebody out of the blue. Choose a book you wouldn't normally read. Give your brain new pathways so that it gets used to change and the unpredictable. Most of our thinking is stuck, so it's freeing to give ourselves a shakeup. This process opens you up to new discoveries, new possibilities.

8. **Resolve Negative Emotions**
Shift negativity by changing your focus.
If you harbour resentment, it will come back to bite you. Resentment is a seed of negativity in your energy field that grows quickly and acts as a magnet to attract other negativity. Don't maintain a vibration that attracts negativity or blaming others; instead, find the reasons you attracted those hurtful situations into your life.

9. **Best Wishes**
Wish the very best for people in your mind and heart.
This will build great karma and energy for you to receive your answers and desires. We are all connected. When you wish the best for others, you wish the best for yourself.

10. Cleanse Your Body
Rest, exercise, hydrate, eat well and immerse yourself in nature.
If your body contains toxins, it will attract toxic emotions and situations in your life. Smoking, alcohol, and drugs need to be eliminated. Eat well and cleanse your body with suitable foods to remove heavy metals and other substances that negatively impact your wellbeing and energy. Exercise regularly (Including yoga and meditation) to maintain a strong physical body and mind.

11. Feel Gratitude
Be thankful and appreciative of what is working for you.
The universe wants to answer you and give you more of the same. What motivates you to help someone? It's a person who is appreciative, grateful, and genuinely sincere. You want people on your side, desiring to help you in any way possible and the universe operates exactly same way. Be thankful.

CONCLUSION

Thank you for allowing me to be part of your journey.

I would love to meet you in person. And so, along with the release of this book, I am introducing a two-day, Freeing Women Workshop, to take the learnings of this book to the next level and magnify the benefits with other like-minded women. Learn more in the next Resources section or visit http://marisarusso.com/events/

I wish you love and best wishes on your healing journey.

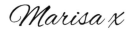

RESOURCES:
STAYING CONNECTED

SOCIAL MEDIA

No matter where I work, I find the same problems. Women in the world feel isolated, alone, and unsupported. For these reasons, I encourage them to join with thousands of women in our private Forensic Healing Facebook group to access ongoing support and encouragement. That includes you! Here is the link to our group:

https://www.facebook.com/groups/ForensicHealing/

This global support system is a place where women share extraordinary stories of healing from working with the Forensic Healing System. You can feel safe and nurtured as I keep a close watch on posts, offering encouragement wherever I can. The stories posted are inspiring, uplifting, empowering, and healing. And as you'd expect, the group is full of great vibes and plenty of sisterly lovin'. I invite you to stay connected and experience this freedom and joy for yourself.

Please 'like' our Forensic Healing Facebook Page
https://facebook.com/forensichealing/

WORKSHOPS

Freeing Women Workshop (Online Video Course coming soon)

Want to take your healing journey to a new level? Join me for two days moving through the 25 step program from this book and much, much more.

http://marisarusso.com/events/

Forensic Healing Diploma (7-Day Workshop or Online Video Course)

A natural therapy system that combines a forensic science approach with intuition to release pain, stress and long term conditions fast. Forensic investigators have one of the most thorough methods to solve crimes. That's why we designed Forensic Healing to use a structured approach to find the who, what, where, when and why of a person's condition - relationship stress, financial blocks, health conditions or anything that causes stress or pain in life.

We teach how to gather the clues by reading a person's energy field and apply one of 90+ healing pathways to resolve the condition. Includes five manuals, 32 hours of video instruction, and online membership content. Create your own business as a Forensic Healing practitioner with the potential of becoming an instructor.

http://forensichealing.com/

Forensic Healing Essentials (1-Day Workshop or Video Course)

Helps you get started in Forensic Healing and develop investigative and intuitive skill sets. Discover how to read a person's body and begin using the new entry-level Forensic Healing method.

http://forensichealing.com/events/

FREE RESOURCES

Women Breaking Free eBook

Visit http://marisarusso.com and download the Women Breaking Free eBook. Yes, it's free to download.

Freeing Women Activation

The healing activation reverses the control and the programmed manipulations of women.

http://marisarusso.com/fug-reader/

SELF HEALING VIDEO COURSES

Abundance Download

Consciousness programming for igniting your prosperity. The powerful Forensic Healing 'Abundance Healing Download' which is equivalent to having a new prosperity/abundance software program downloaded in your consciousness for you to become more financially free and successful. The feedback after receiving this fast track process has been nothing short of miraculous.

http://marisarusso.com/healing-courses/

Jaw and Body Healing

Balance and re-align chronic jaw disorders advanced healing system. This course takes you through a calming jaw alignment healing protocol with clear instruction on each of the 40 healing positions along with inspirational pictures, and uplifting music. It is an excellent healing tool for massage therapists, reiki practitioners, energy healers, naturopaths, dentists, chiropractors or anybody who needs to release trauma, pain and stress.

http://marisarusso.com/healing-courses/

Summon the Universe

Nine steps to creating the life you want. Summon the Universe goes far beyond the laws of attraction. It includes areas that have never been addressed before such as karma, sacrifice, and victim mentality. This journey you are about to embark on will show you proven ways to empower yourself. You will understand that you are the creator of everything in your life. You will attract a life of freedom, happiness and joy.

http://marisarusso.com/healing-courses/

Release Negative Life Patterns

Identify and release negative life patterns that are sabotaging your life. The Virtual Healer solution is a revolutionary interactive system that allows you to be your own healer. You have all you need to heal yourself today. You will identify and release negative life patterns that are sabotaging your life and get the tools to target your negative patterns, layer by layer.

http://marisarusso.com/healing-courses/

Forensic Relationships

Discover secrets to why your power is sourced from the relationships you create. Design your life by removing negative imprints from destructive relationships, create new connections and maximize flow.

http://marisarusso.com/healing-courses/

Made in the USA
Charleston, SC
13 November 2016